Science and sporting performance

Science and sporting performance:

Management or manipulation?

EDITED BY
BRUCE DAVIES
Human Performance Laboratory, University of Salford
AND
GEOFFREY THOMAS
Department for External Studies, University of Oxford

CLARENDON PRESS · OXFORD
1982

Oxford University Press, Walton Street, Oxford OX2 6DP
London Glasgow New York Toronto
Delhi Bombay Calcutta Madras Karachi
Kuala Lumpur Singapore Hong Kong Tokyo
Nairobi Dar es Salaam Cape Town
Melbourne Wellington
and associate companies in
Beirut Berlin Ibadan Mexico City

Published in the United States by
Oxford University Press, New York

British Library Cataloguing in Publication Data

Davies, Bruce
Science and sporting performance.
1. Sports medicine
I. Title II. Thomas, Geoffrey
617'.1027 RC1210
ISBN 0-19-857594-7

Library of Congress Cataloging in Publication Data

Main entry under title:
Science and sporting performance.
Includes bibliographies and index.
1. Sports – Physiological aspects. 2. Physical fitness. 3. Doping in sports. I. Davies, Bruce. II. Thomas, Geoffrey (Geoffrey P.) [DNLM: 1. Sports medicine. QT 260 S413]
RC1235.S4 1982 612'.044 82-7996
AACR2

ISBN 0-19-857594-7

Typeset by Oxford Verbatim Limited
Printed in Great Britain
at the University Press, Oxford
by Eric Buckley
Printer to the University

Foreword

B. B. LLOYD, *Chairman of the Health Education Council*

Science claims all phenomena, natural and artificial, for its purview, and its quest is truth. As A. V. Hill very clearly stated in 1924, champion athletes provide the physiologist with a body of highly consistent data, superbly amenable to analysis. It is sad that today, as a result of pharmacological progress and the emergence of special pressures, every athletic achievement is, to a greater or smaller extent, subject to the bleak doubt that drugs may have played a part, but it is heartening that technological advances are rapidly providing methods of detection and analysis that can identify drugs or prove their use. It seems likely that drug abuse by athletes will be virtually eliminated in a very few years, that the pall of drug suspicion will be lifted from our tracks and fields, and that we shall see a reconvergence of the two meanings of 'sporting' – pertaining to athletic achievement, on the one hand, and to honourable, straightforward, and sportsmanlike activity, on the other.

Certain sports, such as those involving translation of the human body horizontally over the periphery of the earth, have been little if at all affected by drugs, and yet their performers have shown vast improvements over the last century, women more so than men. Are these improvements, in running, jumping, swimming, and skating, due to improvements in power output, or to a greater efficiency in power conversion, or indeed both? My own tentative conclusion is that at a given body weight power, not efficiency, is increasing, but the question is by no means settled. Both power and efficiency are affected by training, but they are also a function of genetic equipment, as those who race greyhounds and horses are aware. The notion of applying the methods of the animal breeder to human beings, whether for nationalistic or athletic (I will not write 'sporting') purposes is repellent though not, as we saw from some reports of Nazi aspirations, absolutely beyond the extremes of the political spectrum.

One problem for the owner of a supremely talented physique is the amount of training that has to be devoted to success in competition, for which a serious price has to be paid in terms of time, money, and personal relationships. It seems to me that our scientific knowledge of the cost-benefit assessment of training is still extremely fragmentary, and that the world of exercise physiologists and sports scientists owes it to the world of performers to determine much more precisely the minimum training efforts needed to reach and maintain a desired level of achievement.

I hope very much that this book will stimulate and promote more scientific work into sporting performance, and convince performers and coaches that they can only gain by co-operating with scientists and then incorporating scientific results into their training schedules. It is certain that every scientist working with athletes is greatly privileged, and that every contribution in this book is offered in all humility to those without whose practical dedication to exercise it could not have been written.

Contents

Contributors

Professor R. V. Brooks, Professor of Chemical Endocrinology, St. Thomas's Hospital Medical School, London.

A. Daggett, Sports Council Research Scholar, Human Performance Laboratory, University of Salford.

Dr B. Davies, Senior Lecturer and Director of the Human Performance Laboratory, University of Salford.

Dr C. T. M. Davies, Head of MRC Muscle Physiology Group in the Department of Physiology and Pharmacology, University of Nottingham.

Professor B. Ekblom, Professor of Physiology at the Karolinska Institute, Stockholm.

Professor G. R. Hervey, Professor of Physiology, University of Leeds.

P. Jakeman, Research Fellow, Human Performance Laboratory, University of Salford.

Dr B. B. Lloyd, Chairman of the Health Education Council, former Director of Oxford Polytechnic and Emeritus Fellow of Magdalen College, Oxford. President of the British Association's Biomedical Sciences Section in 1965 and of the General Section in 1980.

Dr M. J. N. McDonagh, Postdoctoral Research Fellow in the Department of Physiology and Pharmacology, University of Nottingham.

Dr M. O'Brien, Anatomist at the Royal College of Surgeons, Dublin.

Dr P. F. Radford, Director of the Department of Physical Education and Recreation, University of Glasgow. Olympic Bronze medalist and former holder of the world record for the 200 m sprint.

Professor R. J. Shephard is Professor of Applied Physiology and Director of the School of Physical and Health Education, University of Toronto.

Dr A. J. Smith is a lecturer at Bowles Outdoor Pursuit Centre, Eridge Green, Tunbridge Wells, Kent.

Dr G. P. Thomas, Deputy Director of the Oxford University Department for External Studies, and Fellow of Linacre College, Oxford. Recorder of the General Section of the British Association in 1980.

Professor H. Thomason, Head of the Department of Physical Education and Sports Science at Loughborough University of Technology.

Dr. C. L. Williams, Senior Research Fellow in the Department of Physical Education and Sports Science, Loughborough University of Technology.

Introduction

B. DAVIES AND G. P. THOMAS

Sport has long been a crucial element in the culture of most peoples; that it should occupy an increasingly important place in the social life of the more affluent nations is hardly surprising – as preoccupations with survival and the basic necessities of life have receded, so interest has inevitably grown in a wide variety of leisure pursuits including sport. The role which sport now plays is, however, complex and many-sided: it can be seen as the handmaiden of health and physical well-being, as a promoter of social interaction, as a means of individual self-expression, and as a safety-valve in an increasingly pressurized society. The principal definitions of 'sport' in the *Oxford English Dictionary* include the following: 'Pleasant pastime; entertainment or amusement; recreation, diversion'; also 'Participation in games or exercises especially those of an athletic character or pursued in the open air; such games or amusements collectively'. These definitions stress the idea of sports as amusing, diverting, and recreational pastimes – an extension into adult life of the 'play' and 'games' of childhood.

However, sport is also associated with such ideas as 'competition', 'contest', and 'conflict'; with 'winning', 'losing', and 'prizes'. Quite apart from the professionalization of almost all sports, increasing emphasis on the combative as against the recreational aspects of sport has also resulted in many sports being seen as defenders of national prestige (not simply pride) and as instruments of political ideology. There is surely some special irony to be ascribed to the importance sporting prowess has assumed, together with defence and science and technology, in international posturing; alongside the arms 'race' and the space 'race', what? – the sporting performance 'race'?

It was against the background of this ambivalent attitude to sport that the British Association for the Advancement of Science chose to look, in the year of the controversial 1980 Olympic Games, at some aspects of the relations between sport and science, that other dominant ingredient in our culture. It was hoped that a discussion of the convergence, or at least of the points of contact, between sport and science, would prove timely and interesting. A full programme was therefore arranged as part of the Association's Annual Meeting at Salford University in September 1980, under the Presidency of Dr Brian Lloyd, whose distinguished work in human physiology and sports science made him an admirably well-informed Chairman.

The contributions to this volume are, for the most part, based on the papers presented at the meeting, and represent, in the best traditions of the British Association, reports on original work alongside wide-ranging reviews of the subject.

Just as sport itself can be seen in many different lights, so the impact of science and its products on sport can be regarded as desirable, undesirable, or neutral. Investigations of the physiology of the human body and the factors which control and limit its performance are parts of the proper concern of science. From a fuller understanding of these factors springs the possibility of adapting training regimes and techniques so as to improve performance. But at what point does legitimate 'management' become foolhardy (or unfair) manipulation? This question is difficult to resolve in many cases, but the contributions to this volume clarify some of the issues and give us a background against which value judgements may be made.

Scientists involved in exercise physiology are continually seeking ways to make their research applicable. In Chapter 1 Clyde Williams reviews an area which has certainly influenced the performances of endurance events. He describes the metabolism of glycogen and fats, and the influence of training on the utilization of these fuels. The interaction of diet and exercise on glycogen repletion and super compensation are discussed, with possible mechanisms for improved performance.

One of the crucial questions for any sportsman must be what limits his ability to sustain performance, and causes the onset of fatigue. C. T. M. Davies and M. J. N. McDonagh identify the points in the physiological and psychological control system at which fatigue may occur and from which a decrement in performance will result. Concentrating on fatigue in muscle, they show how dependent this is on the intensity of the exercise involved.

Bruce Davies and Philip Jakeman examine the interrelationship between maximal oxygen consumption, running economy, and that controversial topic, the inflection point of lactic acid, commonly known as the anaerobic threshold. They present the results of an experiment investigating the effects of athletic training on these variables and discuss possible implications for future training schedules.

The chapter by Professor Bjorn Ekblom reviews one of the most contentious alleged developments in performance manipulation – so-called 'blood-doping'. He describes basic work, carried out in his own laboratory and elsewhere, on the changes in maximal aerobic capacity caused by variations in haemoglobin concentration resulting from the withdrawal and subsequent reinfusion of blood from the subject's system. Although the extent, if any, to which blood-doping is practised in sport is not known, Ekblom's review suggests that this sort of manipulation does have real implications for sport. This would seem to be a good example of how the results of physiological experiments suggest new ways for the unscrupulous competitor to gain unfair advantage over his fellows; this is doubtless the reasons for Ekblom's 'regret' in reporting his conclusions.

Moira O'Brien, Bruce Davies, and Anne Daggett consider the advantages and disadvantages which arise from the innate anatomical and physiological characteristics of sportsmen and women. They review the current literature with particular reference to the problems of menstruation, and the physiological and biochemical influences on females engaged in high level sport.

Alan Smith's chapter introduces the scope of the rapidly-developing field of biomechanics in sport. Using principles and techniques drawn from mechanical engineering this has enabled fruitful analyses to be made of the human body and its modes of motion. It has also been applied to changes and improvements in equipment design, and the interaction between the equipment and the sportsman. One sport to which this science has made enormous contributions is skiing, and the chapter outlines the remarkable degree of attention which has been paid to the mechanics of skis, bindings, ski–snow interaction, and safety factors.

Brian Lloyd, who achieved the rare distinction of being the President of a Section of the British Association for a second time, presents a fascinating analysis of the factors which influence athletic performance, especially running, and how these factors may be used to produce equations of which some of the parameters have changed over the last century. Extrapolation of these trends facilitates speculations on future performances. It will be interesting to see how these mathematical 'predictions' withstand the test of time. Will there be a biochemical, physiological, or technical development that will substantially influence the parameters?

Professor Harry Thomason records the sad history of drug-taking in sport, in which cycling seems to have blazed the rather unenviable trail. Despite the legislation and associated testing procedures that were eventually introduced by most governing bodies, the hope which was entertained at the end of the 1960s that the practice was under control proved premature. For around that time it became clear that the use of 'anabolic' steroids was becoming common among top-class athletes. Whereas extremely sensitive methods of detecting this dubious practice are now available, notably those stemming from Professor Brooks' work which is described later, Professor Thomason suggests that only radical changes in attitudes within sport can halt the approach of the Pharmaceutical Games.

Until these changes in attitude are adopted there can be no doubt that the most effective way of controlling the use of drugs is to ban them and to police the ban by effective methods of detection and sanction. Professor Raymond Brooks concentrates on techniques for detecting steroid use by athletes. He shows how synthetic 'anabolic' steroids have been tracked down – initially those which are orally-active, then the use of injected steroids – the methods of detecting the latter predating their widespread use by athletes. The novel problem of detecting the administration of the natural male hormone testosterone is being tackled presently and Professor Brooks describes some preliminary work exploring how this may be achieved.

Professor Romane Hervey has been concerned with investigating the actual effects of the so-called 'anabolic' steroids whose use by athletes was based on the believed muscle-building properties of testosterone and hence of related synthetic steroids. Although experiments with rats failed to confirm these premises on which the use of 'anabolic' steroids by humans had been based, further work with human subjects did point to increased muscularity and body weight. Hervey questions whether the effects of steroid drug-taking on athletic performance have been as marked as has sometimes been suggested. He points out that the increased bulk does not arise through the addition of normal muscle, and the effect on muscle performance is unclear. Hervey suggests that the effect of 'anabolic' steroids is rather indirect, for example through enabling more training to be done by reducing muscle fatigue. The harmful effects to which he also refers include abnormal appearance, suppression of natural testosterone secretion, and liver damage.

Peter Radford, perhaps taking advantage of his own experience as a world-class athlete, reports on a pilot survey of contemporary British athletes' views of the role of sports science. His work suggests that British athletes are well aware of the benefits sports science can bring but feel at a definite disadvantage compared with their foreign counterparts in terms of the number and accessibility of sports scientists in this country. However the responses elicited by his questionnaire also indicate something of an equivocal attitude towards sports science in general, the negative aspect stemming from a belief that the presence of sports scientists tends to reduce the pleasurable aspects of sport and make it more of a business.

What of the future? Drawing extensively on recent and current developments, which have seen the increasing application of all branches of science to athletic performance, Professor Roy Shephard paints a disturbing picture of the growing tension between investigators seeking to expand knowledge, and political mentors who seek 'practical' information that can be 'used' in bettering competitive results. Faced with the increasing politicization of sport, the scientist can expect to see the results of his work ruthlessly exploited and the minds and bodies of competitors dangerously manipulated in the cause of political ideology or national prestige. Professor Shephard reviews some of the ways by which this bleak prospect may be lightened, but suggests that ultimately only through reassertion of the Olympic Ideal, with a fuller development of values and beliefs by athlete and scientist together, may a path be found to healthier competition.

It is a pleasure to acknowledge the considerable help we have received from Brian Lloyd, from Don Masterson, Chairman of the Department of Physical Education, Salford University, and from the Oxford University Press. We are naturally greatly indebted to all the contributors – whilst the views expressed are entirely their own, the responsibility for their ordering in this volume has been ours. We are also extremely grateful to Beckman, RIIC Ltd., for their generous help in sponsoring the original meeting.

1 Dietary manipulation and athletic performance

CLYDE WILLIAMS

Introduction

Exercise produces a significant challenge to energy metabolism and results in increased rates of mobilization of the two main metabolic fuels, fat and carbohydrate. The relative contributions of fat and carbohydrate to muscle metabolism received attention as long ago as the late nineteenth century. Chauveau (1887) investigated the arterio-venous differences for oxygen, carbon dioxide, glucose, and fat in the levator muscle of the upper lip of a horse; muscle metabolism was increased simply by allowing the horse to chew. As a result of these studies, Chauveau and colleagues concluded that glucose was the immediate substrate for muscle metabolism. Although there was evidence for a contribution from blood-borne fat, it was believed that fat was a precursor for glycogen formation, within the muscle (Zierler 1976). The idea that carbohydrate, in the form of glucose, was the exclusive metabolic fuel during exercise persisted into the early 1920s, in spite of the available evidence to the contrary (Fletcher and Hopkins 1916; Hill 1926). Whole body respiratory exchange ratios (*R*) for human subjects in different dietary states pointed to the important contribution of fat, as well as carbohydrate, as an energy substrate during exercise (Zuntz 1901, quoted by Gollnick 1977; Anderson and Lusk 1917; Cathcart and Burnett 1925; Krogh and Lindhard 1920; Marsh and Murlin 1928). Furthermore, subsequent animal studies investigating the arterio-venous differences in oxygen and carbon dioxide across working muscles in the anaesthetized dog, showed that the local respiratory quotient (RQ) was less than unity (Himwich and Rose 1927). Fritz Davis, Holtrop and Dundee (1958) were amongst the first to report evidence which showed that fatty-acid oxidation occurs in both resting and in active muscle. Thus these workers were able to provide evidence to support the whole-body respiratory exchange ratio (*R*) studies, which had earlier shown that carbohydrate was not the exclusive fuel during exercise and that fat contributed significantly to muscle metabolism.

The groundwork for our present knowledge of fat and carbohydrate metabolism during exercise was laid by the early studies of Krogh and Lindhard (1920) and Christensen and Hansen (1939). They followed the changes in the respiratory exchange ratios of their subjects during exercise of various intensities and during exercise after different diets. They concluded that:

(1) the proportion of energy utilized during exercise, which was derived from carbohydrate, was larger the heavier the work load;
(2) individuals who consumed carbohydrate-rich diets utilized a larger proportion of carbohydrate during exercise than those living on high-fat diets;
(3) exercise endurance was significantly less in individuals living on high-fat diets and greater in individuals living on high-carbohydrate diets;
(4) during prolonged exercise the contribution of fat to muscle metabolism increased in parallel with the exercise duration.

These conclusions have stood the test of repeated examinations and they have been confirmed and extended over the succeeding years (Jansson 1980).

Fat metabolism

Fat is stored in adipose tissue cells in the form of triglycerides, i.e. a combination of three long-chain fatty acids bound to a glycerol molecule. The free fatty acids (FFA) are mobilized from the triglycerides in adipose tissue cells by the enzymatic cleavage of the triglyceride molecules, which is under hormonal control (Gollnick, Soule, Taylor, Williams, and Ianuzzo 1970). Fatty acids are transported from adipose tissue cells to working muscles in loose combination with plasma albumins, and their extraction by muscle is proportional to their plasma concentration (Armstrong, Steele, Altszuler, Dunn, Bishop, and Debodo 1961; Hagenfeldt and Wahren 1971). During the prolonged, low-intensity exercise fat metabolism can almost completely cover the energy requirements of the working muscles (Havel, Naimark, and Borchgrevink 1963; Young, Shapira, Forrest, Adachi, Lim, and Pelligra 1967; Ahlborg, Felig, Hagenfeldt, Hendler, and Wahren 1974).

Muscle contains fatty acids in the form of lipid droplets of triglycerides which are scattered throughout the sacroplasm of each fibre (Fig 1.1). Intramuscular triglycerides have been suggested as a source of FFA to cover the deficit between the total amount of fat used by the working muscle and the contribution from the oxidation of plasma FFA (Carlson, Ekelund and Fröberg, 1971; Wahren 1973). It has also been suggested that FFA extracted by muscle are converted into triglycerides which act as transitory storage sites of FFA prior to their oxidation in the mitochondria (Zierler 1976). However, it does appear that the immediate fate of the plasma FFA in muscle, whether it is immediate oxidation or temporary storage as triglycerides, is largely dictated by the exercise intensity (Therriault, Beller, Smoake, and Hartley 1973).

The advantages of fat as a fuel during exercise is that the energy yield per unit weight is considerably greater than that obtained from carbohydrate

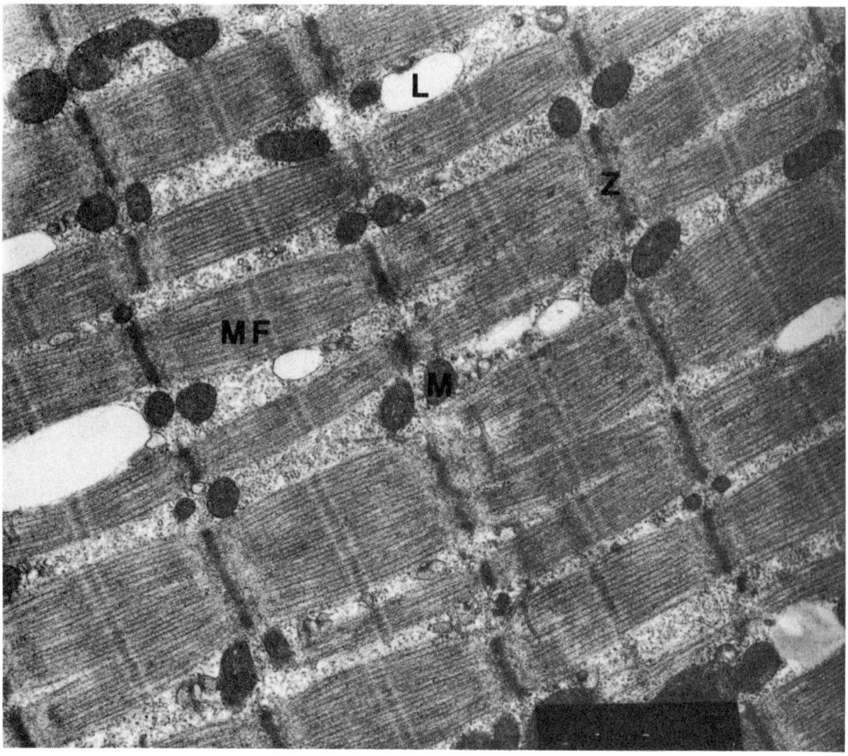

Fig. 1.1. Electron micrograph of a longitudinal section of human vastus lateralis muscle obtained with a needle biopsy. Mitochondria (M) and lipid droplets (L), which are mainly triglycerides, are showed interspersed between the myofibrils (MF). The Z lines (Z) divide the myofibrils into sarcomers. Glycogen granules are dispersed abundantly throughout the intermyofibillar spaces. Magnification × 7500.

metabolism. For example, the complete oxidation of 1 mmol of palmitic acid, a long-chain fatty acid, would yield 129 mmol of ATP, whereas the complete oxidation of 1 mmol of glucose yields 37 mmol of ATP.

Fat is stored in abundance and it accounts for approximately 10 per cent of the body weight of lean males and approximately 15 per cent of the body weight of lean females. The disadvantage of fat as a metabolic fuel during high intensity exercise is that its inherent energy can only be released by oxidation. Fatty-acid oxidation requires more oxygen than the oxidation of an equivalent amount of carbohydrate. Thus the energy yield per litre of oxygen, which is all important during high intensity exercise, is greater when carbohydrate rather than fat is being consumed. The energy yield per litre of oxygen is 5 Kilo calories (21 Kilo joules) from carbohydrate metabolism and 4.7 Kcal (19.7 KJ) from fat metabolism.

Carbohydrate metabolism

Liver glycogen

Carbohydrate is stored in the liver and in skeletal muscles in the form of a polymer of glucose called glycogen. The adult liver, weighing approximately 1.8 kg, contains about 100 g of glycogen, whereas the glycogen concentration of resting skeletal muscle is between 1.0 and 1.5 g/kg of muscle. Analysis of the glycogen concentrations of different tissues involves degradation of glycogen to glucose and then the determination of the resulting glucose concentration. Thus the glycogen concentration of a tissue, such as skeletal muscle, is more usually described in terms of mmol of glucosyl units per kg of muscle (either wet weight or dry weight). Using this latter and more current method of expressing glycogen concentrations, then the values for resting skeletal muscle would be in the range of 60–100 mmol glucosyl units per kg wet weight, whereas the mean value for liver glycogen, after an overnight fast is of the order of 300 mmol of glycosyl units per kg wet weight (Nilsson and Hultman 1973). The main responsibility of liver glycogen is to provide glucose for brain metabolism by ensuring a normal blood glucose concentration under a wide variety of conditions.

In resting man the brain utilizes approximately 120 g of glucose per day, which represents about two-thirds of the glucose released by the liver (Levine and Haft 1970; Newsholme and Start 1973). A decrease in blood glucose concentration below its normal value of between 5.0 mmol/l and 5.6 mmol/l (90 mg per cent and 100 mg per cent) affects the central nervous system and leads to personality changes such as irritability, lethargy, and eventually a hypoglycaemic coma (Levine and Hart 1970). Thus a large decrease in blood glucose concentration during endurance competitions can have a negative influence on the attitude of the athlete towards sustained high-intensity exercise. When liver glycogen is degraded to produce glucose units, the penultimate step involves the conversion of a phosphorylated glucose (glucose 6-phosphate) to free glucose, in the presence of the enzyme glucose 6-phosphatase. Skeletal muscle does not contain glucose 6-phosphatase and so the glucose 6-phosphate formed from glycogen is further degraded to pyruvate by the process known as glycogenolysis (or glycolysis when glucose is the starting-point). Glycogen metabolism does, however, make an indirect contribution to blood glucose homeostatis by providing the liver with precursors for glycogen resynthesis. The metabolites from glycogenolysis, namely lactate, pyruvate, and alanine (Fig 1.2) are transported from skeletal muscle to the liver where they undergo glycogen resynthesis (gluconeogenesis), which is essentially a reversal of glycogenolysis (Newsholme and Start 1973). Liver glycogen contributes to the carbohydrate metabolism of skeletal muscle during exercise via the blood glucose, and the proportional contribution of blood glucose to muscle metabolism

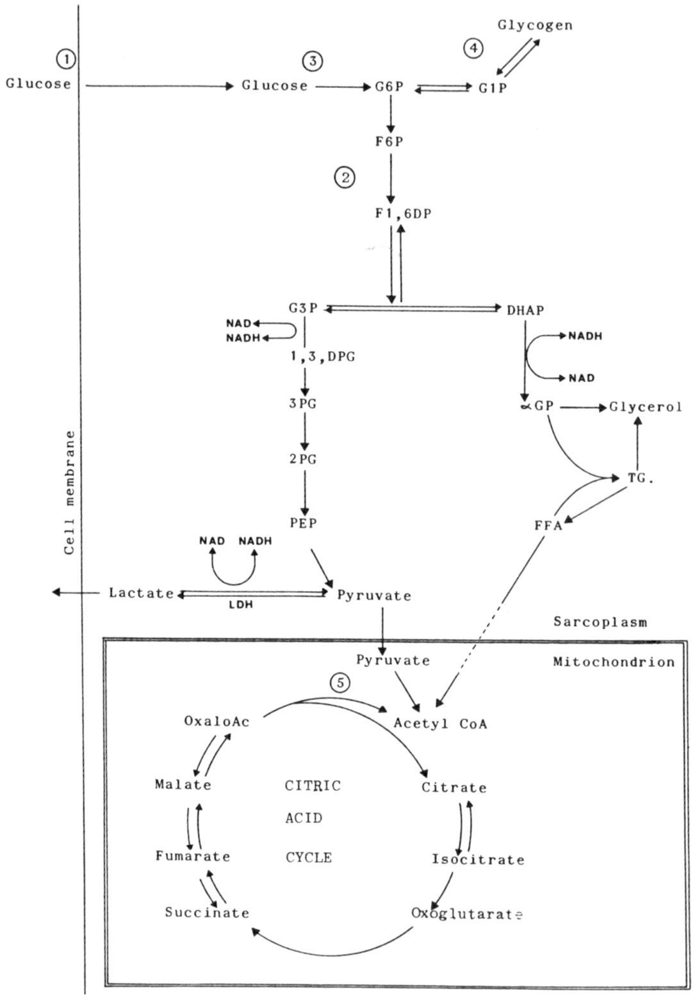

Fig. 1.2. The metabolic pathways of glycolysis and glycogenolysis in muscle. The numbers indicate the various points at which the rates of glycolysis and glycogenolysis can be controlled: (1) glucose entry into the cell; (2) conversion of fructose 6-phosphate to fructose-1,6-diphosphate by the enzyme phosphofructokinase; (3) phosphorylation of glucose by the enzyme hexokinase; (4) glycogen degradation by the enzyme phosphorylase; (5) conversion of pyruvate to acetyl COA by the enzyme pyruvate dehydrogenase.

Glycolytic intermediates: G 6-P, glucose 6-phosphate; G 1-P, glucose 1-phosphate; F 6-P, fructose-6-phosphate; F-1,6-DP, fructose-1,6-diphosphate; G 3-P, glyceraldehyde 3-phosphate; 2-PG, 2-phosphoglycerate; PEP, phospho-enol-pyruvate; DHAP, dihydroxyacetone phosphate; α GP, α glycerophosphate; NAD, nicotinamide-adenine dinucleotide; NADH, nicotinamide-adenine dinucleotide, reduced form; LDH, lactate dehydrogenase; TG, triglycerides.

increases in parallel with the duration of the exercise (Wahren, Felig, Ahlborg, and Jorfeldt 1971). Blood glucose is not freely available for muscle metabolism during exercise, probably because of the reduction in plasma insulin concentration and the inhibition of the glucose phosphorylating enzyme, hexokinase, which occurs as a result of an increase in glucose 6-phosphate concentration at the start of exercise (Newsholme and Start 1973; Galbo, Richter, Hilsted, Holst, Christensen, and Henriksson 1977).

Muscle glycogen

The carbohydrate store in muscle is distributed throughout the muscle cell as granules of glycogen and so it is not as localized as the lipid droplets of triglycerides (Fig 1.1). The advantage of glycogen as a fuel for working muscles is that glycogenolysis and glycolysis can proceed in the absence of an adequate rate of oxygen transport or oxygen utilization (Newsholme and Start 1973). During high-intensity exercise, the rate rather than the capacity for energy resynthesis is all important. Fatigue during exercise, manifest as a reduction in an athlete's speed, reflects the inability of muscle metabolism to match the rate of adenosine 5′-triphosphate (ATP) utilization with an equivalent rate of ATP resynthesis. At the start of high-intensity exercise, ATP resynthesis is covered by the high energy creatine phosphate store within the muscle. In resting muscle the concentration of creatine phosphate is of the order of 60–80 mmol/kg (dry weight) whereas the concentration of ATP is approximately five times less, i.e. 16–20 mmol/kg (dry weight). The high energy creatine phosphate store is almost depleted during the first 30 seconds of high intensity exercise (Karlsson 1971). After the first 5–10 seconds of high intensity exercise the ATP resynthesis from creatine phosphate is complimented to an ever increasing extent by glycogenolysis (Gollnick and Hermansen 1973). Thus, as the creatine phosphate concentration decreases, so there is an increase in the concentration of lactate, as anaerobic glycogenolysis takes over the responsibility of resynthesizing ATP in the working muscles. The increased rate of lactic acid production is not necessarily due to the lack of sufficient oxygen for muscle metabolism, but is probably due to the imbalance between the rates of pyruvate formation by glycogenolysis and pyruvate oxidation by the citric acid cycle (Keul, Doll, and Keppler 1967; Graham, Sjøgaard, Löllgen and Saltin 1978; Holloszy and Booth, 1976). Lactate formation from pyruvate allows glycogenolysis to continue by regenerating the necessary co-factor NAD (nicotin adenine dinucleotide) (Fig 1.2). Although glycogenolysis produces only 3 mmol of ATP per mmol of glucose 6-phosphate, compared with 38 mmol of ATP when complete oxidation occurs, this smaller yield of energy is produced rapidly and frequently (McGilvery 1975).

The disadvantage of having energy production supported almost exclusively by glycogenolysis is that the increase in lactic acid concentration gradually inhibits the glycogenolytic process, and hence its own formation (Newsholme and Start 1973). The increase in hydrogen ion concentration has an inhibitory influence on the enzyme phosphofructokinase (Fig. 1.2), which is one of the controlling enzymes in glycogenolysis. Thus, high rates of carbohydrate metabolism become self-limiting and can therefore only support ATP resynthesis for relatively short periods of time (Gollnick and Hermansen 1973).

Whereas fatigue during short periods of high-intensity exercise is mainly due to the accumulation of hydrogen ions in working muscles, fatigue during prolonged heavy exercise is associated with the depletion of muscle glycogen (Ahlborg, Bergström, Brohult Ekelund, Hultman, and Mashio 1967; Hermansen, Hultman, and Saltin 1967; Gollnick, Ianuzzo, Williams, and Hill 1969; Karlsson and Saltin 1971). The rate of ATP utilization and hence resynthesis during prolonged high-intensity exercise, e.g. long-distance running, is such that the majority of glycogen degradation occurs aerobically and the lactate overflow from pyruvate formation is relatively modest (Costill and Fox 1969). As exercise continues, fatty acid oxidation makes an ever increasing contribution to muscle metabolism. However the continued contribution of glycogenolysis is necessary in order to maintain the desired level of energy production, which appears not to be possible by fat metabolism alone (Hermansen *et al.* 1967).

Glycogen resynthesis in skeletal muscles appears to be a slow process, requiring between 24 and 48 hours to restore the glycogen concentrations to their pre-exercise values (Bergström and Hultman 1966; Piehl 1974; Piehl, Adolfsson, and Nazar 1974; MacDougall, Ward, Sale, and Sutton 1977). Glycogen resynthesis is most rapid during the first few hours of recovery and occurs irrespective of whether the individuals are fed or are fasting (MacDougall *et al.* 1977; Maehlum, Høstmark, and Hermansen 1977; Maehlum and Hermansen 1978). This immediate post-exercise resynthesis of muscle glycogen is illustrated in Fig. 1.3; the same type of response occurs after exercise in non-diabetic and diabetic human subjects as well as in non-diabetic and diabetic animals (Hermansen, Vaage, Williams, Helland, and Nilsen 1975; Maehlum *et al.* 1977; Chen, Ianuzzo, and Williams 1977). Blood glucose and even muscle lactate have been suggested as the immediate substrates for the early resynthesis of muscle glycogen (Hermansen and Vaage 1977; Maehlum and Hermansen 1978).

Diet

The influence of dietary modification of carbohydrate intake and its effect on exercise capacity in human subjects was studied by Christensen and Hansen over 40 years ago (Christensen and Hansen 1939). They reported that exercise time to exhaustion was reduced to below control values when

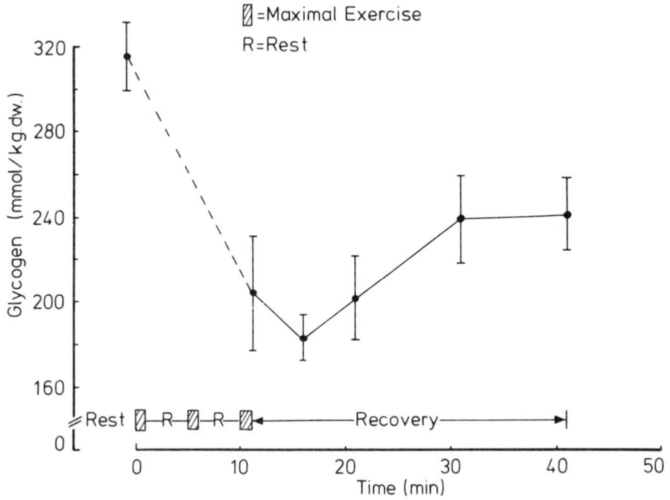

Fig. 1.3. Muscle glycogen concentrations of four subjects before and immediately after three 60-second periods of maximal exercise on a bicycle ergometer. The resting recovery period between each exercise period was four minutes and 30 minutes after the completion of the three bouts of exercise. (Hermansen *et al.* 1975.)

their subjects consumed a low-carbohydrate diet, i.e. mainly fat and protein, for 3–4 days after the control experiment. However, when the exercise experiment was repeated by the same subjects after having consumed a mainly carbohydrate diet for 3–4 days, their exercise time to exhaustion was significantly greater than that recorded for the control experiment, i.e. when the subjects had exercised following several days on a normal mixed diet. This early study highlighted the importance of dietary carbohydrate in preparation for endurance exercise. The more recent studies of Bergström and Hultman (1966) showed that when a carbohydrate-rich diet is fed to individuals after a period of glycogen-depleting exercise, glycogen repletion continues during the following days and increases the glycogen stores of muscle and liver above their pre-exercise values (Bergström and Hultman 1966; Nilsson and Hultman 1973). This glycogen supercompensation phenomenon has been further investigated in an attempt to determine the combination of exercise and dietary modifications necessary to produce the greatest increase in muscle glycogen concentrations (Ahlborg, *et al.* 1967; Hultman 1967). Glycogen supercompensation or carbohydrate loading was found to be most pronounced when the following exercise and dietary manipulations were used; glycogen depletion was produced by prolonged heavy exercise lasting longer than an hour and this was followed by three days on a low-carbohydrate diet, i.e. mainly fat and protein, thereafter the diet was changed to one which was high in carbohydrate for three days.

Exercise was often performed during the low carbohydrate phase of the regime to ensure that muscle glycogen concentration remained low prior to the high carbohydrate phase of the dietary manoeuvre. The exact mechanism responsible for this supercompensation phenomenon has yet to be completely explained. The activity of the glycogen synthetase enzyme complex, in muscle, is inversely related to the muscle glycogen concentration during the immediate post-exercise period; however, glycogen synthesis continues long after the activity of the synthetase enzymes have returned to their pre-exercise values (Adolfsson and Ahren 1971; Bergström, Hultman, and Roch-Norlund 1972).

Endurance capacity is enhanced during exercise following the glycogen loading procedure. Laboratory experiments involving exercise on bicycle ergometers have shown increases in exercise-time to exhaustion of between 38 and 56 per cent (Ahlborg *et al.* 1967; Bergström, Hermansen, Hultman, and Saltin, 1967; Williams, Maughan, Kelman Campbell, and Hepburn 1976). This raises the obvious question of whether or not the glycogen-loading dietary procedure can help to improve speed as well as endurance. In the only reported study involving an endurance race (19 miles) glycogen-loading before the race improved the performance times of the subjects by an average of eight minutes or 5.6 per cent (Karlsson and Saltin 1971). In this study, the speed of the subjects during the early part of the race did not increase after glycogen-loading, but they were able to sustain their optimal pace for longer during the latter part of the race. A closer examination of the results of this study reveals that the subjects could be divided into two groups, one group having higher maximum oxygen-uptake values and faster race times than the other group. This first group was made up of experienced distance runners whereas the second group were active physical education students. The reduction in the running time for the 19 miles, was five minutes (3.2 per cent) and 12 minutes (7.6 per cent) for the first and second groups of runners respectively. The endurance runners had higher concentrations of muscle glycogen than the second group of subjects, and this may partly explain the differences in race times before and after the glycogen-loading procedures. The higher glycogen concentrations of the trained runners, without dietary modification, probably allowed them to sustain their optimal pace for more or less the entire race, hence the contribution of the dietary manipulation procedure was less effective for these individuals.

In a more recent study the carbohydrate-loading procedure was reported to improve treadmill running time to exhaustion by 9 per cent (Goforth, Hodgdon, and Hilderbrand 1980). The running speeds for the nine well-trained individuals were equivalent to 80 per cent of their maximum oxygen-uptake values. Although the carbohydrate-loading procedure increased the average running time to exhaustion from 120 minutes to 130 minutes, there was considerable interindividual variation in running performance (Goforth, personal communication). The dietary manipulation was well controlled in this study and the isocaloricity of each diet was achieved by use of a combination of liquid and solid foods. Unfortunately the changes in muscle glycogen concentrations were not determined, and so the efficacy of the dietary procedure in elevating the glycogen stores of the muscle could not be judged. The daily energy intake of these subjects was 8.37 MJ/day (3500 Kcal/day), of which 46 per cent was carbohydrate, 42 per cent was fat and 12 per cent was protein, whereas on the high-carbohydrate diet the proportions of carbohydrate, fat and protein were 64, 24, and 12 per cent respectively.

When athletes attempt to use the dietary and exercise procedure in order to enhance their endurance performance, their lack of success in achieving greater endurance may be due to an inadequate carbohydrate intake. When the weighed food intake of a group of athletes was recorded during their attempt to achieve glycogen supercompensation, in preparation for different endurance events, considerable interindividual variation existed in their ability to consume large quantities of carbohydrate (Wootton, Shorten, and Williams 1981). The proportion of carbohydrate in their normal diet averaged 43 per cent, whereas on the low- and high-carbohydrate diets they averaged 10 and 55 per cent respectively. Surprisingly, the proportions of carbohydrate consumed on the high-carbohydrate diet ranged from 43–66 per cent and some individuals were unable to increase their carbohydrate intake much above that of their normal diet. How much of this variability is related to the sharp contrast in the composition of the food intake in changing from the low-carbohydrate diet to the high-carbohydrate diet and/or simply the wrong choice of foods, remains to be investigated. The relative proportions of carbohydrate, fat, and protein necessary for a well balanced diet do not appear to be common knowledge within the athletic fraternity. In a survey designed to discover the nutritional knowledge of coaches and athletes, over half of those who participated indicated that the most desirable diet for athletes was one which consisted of 45 per cent carbohydrate, 10 per cent fat and 45 per cent protein (Bentivegna, Kelly, and Kalenak 1979). The idea that the protein intake should be a large proportion of an athlete's daily food intake still persists, in spite of evidence and advice to the contrary (American Dietetic Association 1980).

In addition to the possibility that athletes may misjudge what comprises a balanced diet, there is the greater risk that the large time commitment of employment and training may leave insufficient time for an adequate food intake. Endurance athletes, covering up to a 100 miles per week in training, have to include at least two runs each day in order to achieve this high-mileage. This daily schedule of long runs makes considerable demands on the athlete's glycogen stores, and even with adequate meals there may be

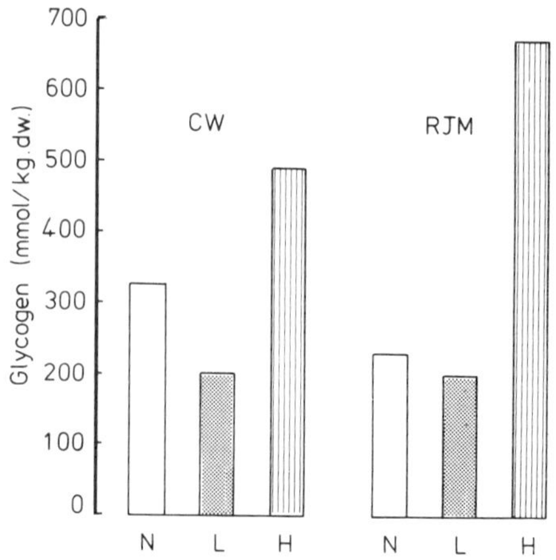

Fig. 1.4. Muscle glycogen concentrations of two subjects during the three phases of the carbohydrate-loading procedure, i.e. after a normal diet (N), after exhaustive exercise and three days on a low-carbohydrate diet (L), and after three days on a high-carbohydrate diet (H). Subject CW had not undertaken heavy exercise on the two days preceding this experiment, whereas the athlete (RJM) had completed a full week of endurance training with a 20 mile run on the day preceding this experiment. (Williams, unpublished.)

insufficient time for resynthesis of muscle glycogen (Costill, Bowers, Branam, and Sparks 1971). This is illustrated in the results of one study of glycogen supercomposition in which one of the subjects was an athlete who ran between 90 and 100 miles per week in training. The pre-exercise muscle glycogen concentrations for an active untrained subject (CW) and for the athlete (RJM) are shown in Fig. 1.4 (Williams, unpublished observations). The athlete had completed a full week of training and did not modify his training on the days preceding the experiment. The low muscle glycogen concentration of the athlete, following his normal diet, was not very much greater than his glycogen concentration after exercise to exhaustion plus three days on a low carbohydrate diet. A combination of a decreased training intensity and a carbohydrate-rich diet was, however, successful in increasing his muscle glycogen concentration. There is then the real possibility that many endurance athletes may not have restored their glycogen stores to their normal values before competition and so begin to compete with a metabolic disadvantage, i.e. low concentrations of muscle glycogen. Recently it has been reported that normal non-supercompensated glycogen stores can be achieved simply by increasing the carbohydrate content of the diet over a 24 hour period. However it appears that the carbohydrate intake should amount to 70 per cent of the daily food intake, and be consumed in two meals during the 24 hour period following glycogen depletion (Sherman, Costill, Fink and Miller 1980).

Training combined with an adequate food intake produces an increase in the concentration of muscle glycogen (Gollnick, Armstrong, Saltin, Saubert, Sembrowich, and Shepherd 1973). This adaptation to endurance training is due to the increased oxidative capacity of skeletal muscles, which therefore have a greater capacity to utilize fatty-acid oxidation to support their energy needs during exercise. This shift towards a greater fat metabolism during high-intensity exercise has a carbohydrate-sparing effect and thus optimizes the utilization rate of muscle glycogen (Holloszy and Booth 1976; Rennie, Winder, and Holloszy 1976; Costill, Coyle, Dalsky, Evans, Fink, and Hoopes 1977). Paradoxically the carbohydrate-loading procedure appears to reverse the training-induced shift towards an increased fat metabolism. Exercise performed after undergoing the carbohydrate-loading procedure relies on a greater amount of carbohydrate metabolism than occurs during exercise after a normal diet (Rennie and Johnson 1974; Williams *et al.* 1976; Maughan, Williams, Campbell, and Hepburn 1978; Jansson 1980). There is some evidence that the size of the glycogen store in muscle may influence its own rate of utilization during exercise (Klausen and Sjøgaard 1980). However, during exercise after the dietary manipulation of carbohydrate intake, the increased carbohydrate metabolism is probably a response to the insulin-induced decrease in fatty-acid mobilization (Rennie and Johnson 1974). The extraction of fatty acids from plasma by muscle is proportional to the arterial concentration of fatty acids, and so a decreased plasma fatty-acid concentration is accompanied by a decreased fatty-acid oxidation and hence an increased carbohydrate metabolism (Hagenfeldt and Wahren 1971).

Pre-exercise ingestion of glucose drinks has also been shown to increase insulin concentrations, decrease fatty-acid concentrations in plasma, and increase the rate of glycogen utilization during exercise (Costill *et al.* 1977; Galbo, Holst, and Christensen 1979). Although the pre-competition meal should be mainly carbohydrate, it should be ingested about three hours before competition so the absorption is completed and insulin concentrations have returned to their normal values before exercise begins. In this way the risk of upsetting the normal substrate-hormone balance of an athlete before competition is minimized. During endurance events, the ingestion of concentrated glucose solutions should also be avoided because of their slow clearance rates from the gut and their insulinogenic effects. The glucose concentrations of drinks ingested during endurance events have been recommended as no greater than 2.5 g of glucose per 100 ml of water (Fordtran and Saltin 1967; Costill, Kammer, and Fisher 1970; Costill and Saltin 1974). Adequate fluid intake should be ensured both before and during endurance events in order to prevent excessive dehydration and subsequent impairment of performance. It has been recommended that endurance athletes begin increasing their water intake about two hours before competition by ingesting about 600 ml, which is then followed by 400–500 ml approximately 15 minutes before the start of the competition (American Dietetic Association 1980). Carbohydrate-loading has been suggested as having an added advantage in that it helps prevent dehydration during endurance competitions (Sharman 1981). Each gram of glycogen stored in the muscle has approximately 3 g of water stored with it, and this water is released during the gradual depletion of muscle glycogen (Olsen and Saltin 1970). The availability of this water may off-set the dehydration which normally occurs during prolonged exercise and which is associated with an excessive sweat loss.

In conclusion, the currently available evidence suggests that the minimal nutritional preparation of the trained athlete for endurance competitions should include a deliberate increase in carbohydrate intake 2–3 days before competition with an accompanying decrease in training intensity. If the athlete is to attempt the full dietary manipulation in order to achieve glycogen supercompensation, in preparation for a major competition, then it is advisable to rehearse the procedure during training or during the preparation for minor competition early in the season. Ingestion of concentrated glucose drinks immediately before and during endurance competitions does not appear to aid endurance performance, whereas an adequate water intake is necessary in order to avoid dehydration and subsequent failure of performance.

Acknowledgements

The author acknowledges the financial support of The Sports Council and the encouragement of the members of the Sports Science Research Group, Loughborough University of Technology.

References

Adolfsson, S., and Ahren, K. (1971). Control mechanism for the synthesis of glycogen in striated muscle. In *Muscle metabolism during exercise* (eds. B. Pernow, and B. Saltin,) pp. 257–72. Plenum Press, New York.

Ahlborg, B., Bergström, J., Brohult, J., Ekelund, L-G., Hultman, E., and Mashio, G. (1967). Human muscle glycogen content and capacity for prolonged exercise after different diets. *Försvarsmedicin* **3**, 85–99.

—— Felig, P., Hagenfeldt, L., Hendler, R., and Wahren, J. (1974). Substrate turnover during prolonged exercise in man: splanchnic and leg metabolism of glucose, free fatty acids and amino acids. *J. Clin. Invest.* **53**, 1080–90.

American Dietetic Association (1980). Position statement: nutrition and physical fitness. *J. Am. Diet. Ass.* **76**, 437–43.

Anderson, R. J. and Lusk, G. (1917). The inter-relation between diet and body condition and energy production during mechanical work. *J. biol. Chem.* **32**, 421–45.

Armstrong, D. T., Steele, R., Altszuler, N., Dunn, A., Bishop, J. S. and Debodo, R. C. (1961). Regulation of plasma free fatty acid turnover. *Am. J. Physiol.* **201**, 9–15.

Bentivegna, A., Kelly, E. J., and Kalenak, A. (1979). Diet, fitness, and athletic performance. *Physician. Sports Med.* **7**, 99–105.

Bergström, J., Hermansen, L., Hultman, E., and Saltin, B. (1967). Diet, muscle glycogen and physical performance. *Acta. physiol. scand.* **71**, 140–50.

—— and Hultman, E. (1966). Muscle glycogen synthesis after exercise. An enhancing factor localized to muscle cells in man. *Nature, Lond.* **210**, 309–10.

—— —— and Roch-Norlund, A. E. (1972). Muscle glycogen synthetase in normal subjects: basal values, effect of glycogen depletion by exercise and of a carbohydrate rich diet following exercise. *Scand. J. clin. Lab. Invest.* **29**, 231–6.

Carlson, L. A., Ekelund, L-G, and Fröberg, S. O. (1971). Concentration of triglycerides, phospholipids and glycogen in skeletal muscle and of free fatty acids and β-hydroxbutyric acid in blood in man in response to exercise. *Eur. J. clin. Invest.* **1**, 248–54.

Cathcart, E. P. and Burnett, W. A. (1925). The influence of muscle work on metabolism in varying conditions of diet. *Proc. R. Soc. B* **99**, 405–26.

Chauveau, M. A. (1887). Experiences pour la determination du coefficient de l'activite nutritive et respiratoire des muscles en repos et en travail. *C. R. hebd. Séanc. Acad. Sci. Paris* **104**, 1126–32.

Chen, V., Ianuzzo, C. D. and Williams, C. (1977). Exercise-induced changes in muscle glycogen concentrations in streptozotocin-diabetic rats. *J. Physiol., Lond.* **269**, 59–60P.

Christensen, E. H. and Hansen, O. (1939). Arbeitsfähigket und ehrnährung. *Skand. arch. physiol.* **81**, 160–75.

Costill, D. L. and Fox, E. L. (1969). Energetics of marathon running. *Med. Sci. Sports* **1**, 81–6.

—— and Saltin, B. (1974). Factors limiting gastric emptying during rest and exercise. *J. appl. Physiol.* **37**, 679–83.

—— Bowers, R., Branam, G., and Sparks, K. (1971). Muscle glycogen utilization during prolonged exercise on successive days. *J. appl. Physiol.* **31**, 834–8.

—— Coyle, E., Dalsky, G., Evans, W., Fink, W. and Hoopes, D. (1977). Effects of elevated plasma FFA and insulin on muscle glycogen usage during exercise. *J. appl. Physiol.* **43**, 695–9.

—— Kammer, W. F., and Fisher, A. (1970). Fluid ingestion during long distance running. *Archs. envir. Hlth* **21**, 520–5.

Fletcher, W. M. and Hopkins, F. G. (1916). The respiratory process in muscle and the nature of muscular motion. *Proc. R. Soc. B* **B89**, 444–67.

Fordtran, J. A. and Saltin, B. (1967). Gastric emptying and intestinal absorption during prolonged severe exercise. *J. appl. Physiol.* **23**, 331–5.

Fritz, I., Davis, D. G., Holtrop, R. H., and Dundee, H. (1958). Fatty acid oxidation by skeletal muscle during rest and activity. *Am. J. Physiol.* **194**, 379–86.

Galbo, H., Holst, J. J., and Christensen, N. J. (1979). The effect of different diets and of insulin on the hormonal response to prolonged exercise. *Acta physiol. scand.* **107**, 19–32.

—— Richter, E. A., Hilsted, J., Holst, J. J., Christensen, N. J., and Henriksson, J. (1977). Hormonal regulation during prolonged exercise. *Ann. N. Y. Acad. Sci.* **301**, 72–80.

Goforth, H. W., Jr., Hodgdon, J. A., and Hilderbrand, R. L. (1980). A double blind study of the effects of carbohydrate loading upon endurance performance. *Med. Sci. Sports Exercise* **12**, 108A.

Gollnick, P. D. (1977). Free fatty acid turnover and the availability of substrates as a limiting factor in prolonged exercise. *Ann. N. Y. Acad. Sci.* **301**, 64–71.

—— and Hermansen, L. (1973). Biochemical adaptations to exercise: anaerobic metabolism. In *Exercise and sports science reviews* (ed. J. H. Wilmore,) Vol. 1, pp. 1–43. Academic Press, New York.

—— Armstrong, R. B., Saltin, B., Saubert, C. W., Sembrowich, W. L., and Shepherd, R. E. (1973). Effect of training on enzyme activity and fibre composition of human skeletal muscle. *J. appl. Physiol.* **34**, 107–11.

—— Ianuzzo, C. D., Williams, C., and Hill, T. R. (1969). Effect of prolonged severe exercise on the ultra structure of human skeletal muscle. *Int. Z. angew. Physiol.* **27**, 257–65.

—— Soule, R. G., Taylor, A. W., Williams, C., and Ianuzzo, C. D. (1970). Exercise-induced glycogenolysis and lipolysis in the rat: hormonal influence. *Am. J. physiol.* **219**, 729–33.

Graham, T., Sjøgaard, G., Löllgen, H., and Saltin, B. (1978). NAD in muscle of man at rest and during exercise. *Pflugers Arch. ges. Physiol.* **376**, 35–9.

Hagenfeldt, L. and Wahren, J. (1971). Metabolism of free fatty acids and ketone bodies in skeletal muscle. In *Muscle metabolism during exercise* (eds. B. Pernow and B. Saltin). Plenum Press, New York.

Havel, R. J., Naimark, A., and Borchgrevink, C. F. (1963). Turnover rate and oxidation of free fatty acids of blood plasma in man during exercise: studies during continuous infusion of palmitate-l-C^{14}. *J. clin. Invest.* **42**, 1054–63.

Hermansen, L., Hultman, E., and Saltin, B. (1967). Muscle glycogen during prolonged severe exercise. *Acta physiol. scand.* **71**, 129–39.

—— and Vaage, O. (1977). Lactate disappearance and glycogen synthesis in human muscle after maximal exercise. *Am. J. Physiol.* **233**, E422–29.

—— —— Williams, C., Helland, A., and Nilsen, L. (1975). Glycogen synthesis and lactate metabolism during recovery after maximal exercise in man. *Acta physiol. scand.* **95**, 2.

Hill, A. V. (1926). *Muscular activity*. University Park Press, Baltimore, Md.

Himwich, H. E. and Rose, M. I. (1927). The respiratory quotient of exercising muscles. *Am. J. Physiol.* **81**, 485–6.

Holloszy, J. O. and Booth, F. W. (1976). Biochemical adaptations to endurance exercise in muscle. *Ann Rev. Physiol.* **38**, 273–91.

Hultman, E. (1967). Studies on muscle metabolism of glycogen and active phosphate in man with special reference to exercise and diet. *Scand. J. clin. Lab. Invest., Suppl.,* **19**, 94.

Jannson, E. (1980). Diet and muscle metabolism in man. *Acta physiol. scand., Suppl.,* 487.

Karlsson, J. (1971). Lactate and phosphagen concentration in working muscle of man. *Acta physiol. scand.,* Suppl., 358.

—— and Saltin, B. (1971). Diet, muscle glycogen and endurance performance. *J. appl. Physiol.* **31**, 203–6.

Keul, J., Doll, E., and Keppler, D. (1967). The substrate supply of human skeletal muscle at rest, during and after work. *Experientia* **23**, 974–9.

Klausen, K. and Sjøgaard. (1980). Glycogen stores and lactate accumulation in skeletal muscle of man during intense bicycle exercise. *Scand. J. Sports. Sci.* **2**, 7–12.

Krogh, A. and Lindhard, J. (1920). The relative value of fat and carbohydrate as sources of muscular energy. *Biochem. J.* **14**, 290–363.

Levine, R. and Haft, D. E. (1970). Carbohydrate homeostatis. *New Engl. J. Med.* **283**, 237–46.

MacDougall, J. D., Ward, G. R., Sale, D. G. and Sutton, J. R. (1977). Muscle glycogen repletion after high intensity intermittent exercise. *J. appl. Physiol.* **42**, 129–32.

McGilvery, R. W. (1975). The use of fuels for muscular work. In *Metabolic adaptation to prolonged physical exercise* (eds. H. Howald and J. R. Poortmans). Birkhäuser, Basel, pp. 12–30.

Maehlum, S. and Hermansen, L. (1978). Muscle glycogen concentration during recovery after prolonged severe exercise in fasting subjects. *Scand. J. clin. Lab. Invest.* **38**, 557–60.

—— Høstmark, A. T., and Hermansen, L. (1977). Synthesis of muscle glycogen during recovery after prolonged severe exercise in diabetic and non-diabetic subjects. *Scand. J. clin. Lab. Invest.* **37**, 309–16.

Marsh, M. E. and Murlin, J. R. (1928). Muscular efficiency on high carbohydrate and high fat diets. *J. Nutr.* **1**, 105–37.

Maughan, R. J., Williams, C., Campbell, D. M., and Hepburn, D. (1978). Fat and carbohydrate metabolism during low intensity exercise: effects of the availability of muscle glycogen. *Eur. J. appl. Physiol.* **39**, 7–16.

Newsholme, E. A. and Start, C. (1973). *Regulation in metabolism.* Wiley Interscience, London.

Nilsson, L. and Hultman, E. (1973). Liver glycogen in man – the effect of total starvation or a carbohydrate-poor diet followed by carbohydrate refeeding. *Scand. J. clin. Lab. Invest.* **32**, 325–30.

Olsen, K. E. and Saltin, B. (1970). Variations in total body water with muscle glycogen changes in man. *Acta. physiol. scand.* **80**, 11–18.

Piehl, K. (1974). Time course for refilling of glycogen stores in human muscle fibres following exercise-induced glycogen depletion. *Acta physiol. scand.* **90**, 297–302.

—— Adolfsson, S., and Nazar, K. (1974). Glycogen storage and glycogen synthetase activity in trained and untrained muscle of man. *Acta physiol. scand.* **90**, 779–88.

Rennie, M. J. and Johnson, R. H. (1974). Effects of an exercise–diet program on metabolic changes with exercise in runners. *J. appl. Physiol.* **37**, 821–25.

—— Winder, W. M., and Holloszy, J. O. (1976). A sparing effect of increased free fatty acids on muscle glycogen content in exercising rat. *Biochem. J.* **156**, 647–55.

Sharman, I. M. (1981). Glycogen loading: advantages and possible disadvantages. *Br. J. Sports Med.* **15**, 64–7.

Sherman, W. M., Costill, D. L., Fink, W. J., and Miller, J. M . (1980). Dietary influence on 24 hour muscle glycogen restoration following depletion. *Med. Sci. Sports Exercise* **12**, 127A.

Therriault, D. G., Beller, G. A., Smoake, J. A., and Hartley, L. H. (1973). Intramuscular energy sources in dogs duting physical work. *J. Lipid Res.* **14**, 54–60.

Wahren, J. (1973). Substrate utilization by exercising muscle in man. *Progr. Cardiol.* **2**, 255–80.

—— Felig, P., Ahlborg, G., and Jorfeldt, L. (1971). Glucose metabolism during leg exercise in man. *J. clin. Invest.* **50**, 2715–2725.

Williams, C., Maughan, R. J., Kelman, R. G., Campbell, D. M., and Hepburn, D. (1976). Fat mobilization during exercise following dietary and exercise-induced changes in muscle glycogen. *Proc. Nutr. Sco.* **35**, 135A.

Wootton, S. A., Shorten, M., and Williams, C. (1981). Manipulation of dietary carbohydrate in a carbohydrate-loading regime. *Proc. Nutr. Soc.* **40**, 3A.

Young, D. R., Shapira, J., Forrest, R., Adachi, R. R., Lim, R., and Pelligra, R. (1967). A model for evaluation of fatty acid metabolism for man during prolonged exercise. *J. appl. Physiol.* **23**, 716–725.

Zierler, K. L. (1976). Fatty acids as substrates for heart and skeletal muscle. *Circulation Res.* **38**, 459–63.

2 Central and peripheral mechanisms of muscle fatigue

C. T. M. DAVIES AND M. J. N. McDONAGH

Introduction

Skeletal muscle is said to fatigue when it fails to produce and sustain the required or expected force. The mechanisms controlling muscular force are complex and depend on several physiological and psychological control systems (Fig. 2.1). Fatigue may occur at one or several of the steps illustrated at Fig. 1.1. A major drive in research has been towards identifying at which of these stages fatigue actually occurs. Much of the best information comes from work involving the electrical stimulation of animal and human muscle. There is still uncertainty about the detailed relationship between fatigue under these conditions and fatigue in voluntary contractions of muscle. In maximum voluntary contractions, motor units are usually firing asynchronously, whereas in the stimulated contraction all the motor units are made to fire together.

Central fatigue

In voluntary contractions, part of the fatigue may be due to loss of central motor drive (a loss of will-power or a change in central nervous system mechanisms). There may be a failure to recruit enough motor units to

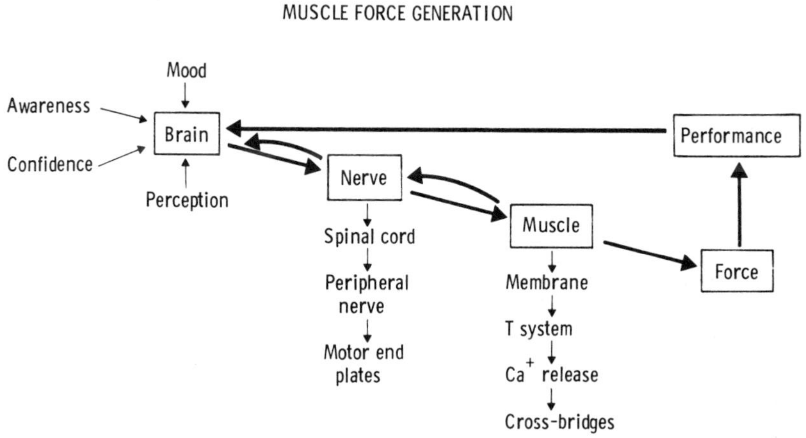

Fig. 2.1. A schematic representation of muscle force generation in man.

sustain the force, or a failure to drive them at sufficiently high frequencies. This type of fatigue is probably less common in top-class sportsmen who are highly motivated, but it does occur in normal healthy subjects. In these subjects it can be shown that even when voluntary force is declining as a result of fatigue, the involuntary force produced by electrical stimulation shows much less fatigue (Ikai, Yabe, and Ishii 1967). Further evidence for central fatigue comes from the work of Asmussen and Mazin (1978) who showed that fatigue can be reduced by giving the subject diverting activities to occupy the mind between bouts of exercise. It may be that a certain amount of the subjective effort required in voluntary contractions is needed to overcome tonic inhibition of motor neurons which has its source in afferent input from sensory receptors. This is the explanation offered by Gandevia and McCloskey (1977) for their experimental observation that objects lifted by the extension of the thumb feel lighter when the thumb is anaesthetized.

Peripheral fatigue

There is no doubt that central fatigue does occur, but it is highly variable and difficult to measure objectively. Fatigue in the peripheral mechanisms (motor nerve axons and muscle cells) is measurable. Voluntary central drive can be bypassed by stimulating the motor axons of muscles electrically to produce muscular force. Using these techniques, it can be shown that the force produced by this stimulation declines following either voluntary exercise or several minutes of electrical stimulation.

The major question is, which of the steps illustrated in Fig. 2.1 is responsible for this peripheral fatigue? It is useful to sketch some of the evidence implicating each step.

Neuro-muscular junction

Krnjevic and Miledi (1958) investigated fatigue effects at the neuromuscular junction using the isolated rat diaphragm. They found that muscle fibres cannot respond for more than a few minutes at frequencies greater than 50/s without intermittent failure of action potentials and eventually complete block. This was found to be due to a reduction in end-plate potential and to an increase in the threshold of the muscle fibre. If excitation was maintained at a frequency of 10/s, the likelihood of propagation failure was small.

Muscle action potential

The best evidence for failure of the muscle action potential in fatigue comes from studies on single frog fibres, in which the muscle-fibre membrane is stimulated directly and neuro-muscular transmission is bypassed (direct stimulation). Luttgau (1965) found that at frequencies of 100 Hz there was intermittent failure of muscle action potentials. In the directly stimulated soleus muscle of the mouse, it was fround that muscle stimulated at frequencies of 100 Hz quickly fatigued, but tension recovered immediately if there was a sudden drop of stimulation frequency to 20 Hz. Stimulation of this isolated muscle in low $[Na^+]$ produced a loss of force similar to that produced by high-frequency stimulation (Jones 1979; Jones, Bigland-Ritchie, and Edwards 1979). In man, this type of failure is likely to occur only at the highest rates of firing (i.e. during near-maximum contractions) or where conditions become anoxic due to ischaemia. Stephens and Taylor (1972) found that the smoothed rectified electromyogram (SRE) fell with the same time course as force during sustained voluntary contractions of human muscle. This parallel fall continued until the force was no longer sufficient to cut off the blood supply to the muscles. At this point the fall in SRE ceased, although the force continued to decline.

It would appear that the body has a mechanism to counteract high frequency fatigue. Marsden, Meadows, and Merton (1976) have demonstrated that in a sustained voluntary contraction the mean firing rate of motor neurons falls progressively with fatigue. In stimulated contractions of human adductor pollicis muscle, it has been found that the electromyogram declines at stimulation rates of 50 Hz but not at 20 Hz (Bigland-Ritchie, Jones, and Woods 1979). In these human experiments it is not possible to say whether the reduction in SRE is due to failure of neuro-muscular transmission or in muscle action potential. Parallel experiments on curarized, directly stimulated isolated mouse muscle produced similar results – thus strongly implicating action potential failure at 50 Hz and above (Bigland-Ritchie *et al.* 1979).

Excitation–contraction coupling

Even at low frequencies of stimulation, at which neuro-muscular function or action potential failure is not a problem, reduction in force still occurs. There is a great deal of evidence to point to a breakdown in excitation-contraction coupling. Excitation–contraction coupling is a general term for several processes transmitting the signal for contracting from the muscle action potential to the actin and myosin filaments. It includes transmission of the action potential along the t-tubular system – transmission by an unknown mechanism from t-system to the sacroplasmic reticulum, release of calcium from the sarcoplasmic reticulum, calcium binding to troponin, and finally the reabsorption of the calcium by the sacroplasmic reticulum.

The best evidence for fatigue in excitation–contraction coupling comes from single frog-muscle fibres stimulated at low frequencies (0.2–5/s)

(Grabowski, Lobsiger, and Luttgau 1972). In these fibres tension declined, but there was little change in the action potentials. However, the application of caffeine (which causes directly, release of calcium from the sacroplasmic reticulum) to fatigued fibres restored twitch tension indicating that the fatigue was in the coupling mechanism, not in the contractile process itself. The exact site of excitation–contraction coupling fatigue is unknown.

It has been shown recently (Dawson, Gadian, and Wilkie 1978), using nuclear magnetic resonance spectroscopy of whole frog muscle, that the decrease of force in fatigued muscle is proportional to the increase in adenosine 5′-pyrophosphate (ADP) and in H^+. At present it is too early to say whether either relation is causal rather than coincidental. A dependence of isometric-force development on [ADP] [H^+] and [Pi] could arise from product inhibition of the contractile system or from interference with the activation of contraction.

Another feature of fatigue is the slowing of relaxation of a tetanus (Edwards, Hill, and Jones 1975). Dawson, Gadian, and Wilkie (1980) have shown that unlike force development, this parameter is linearly related to the affinity for adenosine 5′-triphosphate (ATP) hydrolysis. They argue that this increase in relaxation time is related to a reduced rate of re-uptake of calcium by the sacroplasmic reticulum, possibly due to the inhibition caused by high levels of ADP.

Depletion of energy stores

One obvious source of fatigue involving myosin–actin reactions is a depletion of the energy sources needed for contraction. However, it should be noted that such stores are also needed for excitation–contraction coupling, in particular to fuel the calcium pump involved in the re-uptake of calcium into the sarcoplasmic reticulum.

The immediate energy source used for actin–myosin inter-action and calcium pumping (and for all cellular energetic processes) is ATP. However, the actual levels of ATP in muscle are very low (5–7 μmol/g) (Newsholme 1977). It has to be constantly resynthesized.

The main reaction sequences in the cell producing ATP are:

(1) The Lohmann reaction CrP + ADP→ATP + Cr.
(2) The anaerobic breakdown of glycogen (glycolysis).
(3) The aerobic breakdown of glucose, glycogen, and fatty acids via the Krebs cycle and oxidative phosphorylation.

At the highest rates of work the glycolytic capacity of the muscle cell cannot supply energy at the rate required. Only the formation of ATP from phosphocreatine is fast enough. However, the reserves of phosphocreatine are rapidly exhausted (after about 40 seconds of maximal exercise) and the work rate drops or ceases. For example, following 40–55 seconds of a held maximum voluntary contraction of m. quadriceps femoris in man, phosphocreatine levels dropped to 15–16 per cent of the exercise values. Following exercise, the phosphocreatine recovered to 75 per cent of the exercise values after one minute (Harris, Edwards, Hultman, Nordesjo, Nylind, and Sahlin 1976). Most of this recovery would seem to depend on aerobic metabolism in muscle as it is prevented by an occluded blood supply.

The anaerobic breakdown of glycogen can maintain lower levels of muscular power output for 2–3 minutes in the absence of oxygen (Margaria 1976). This anaerobic breakdown of glycogen leads to a rise in the lactic acid content of muscle, and hence to a rise in $[H^+]$. Once lactate levels rise, recovery from fatigue is prolonged as the reduction in H^+ and lactate levels occurs very slowly. This has a very practical application, whenever strenuous work has to be done. For example, if an athlete training for the 400 m covers the whole distance at his maximum speed he will incur an acidosis which will be removed only after a rest of at least 0.5 hours. In a total of four hours he can, therefore, run at most three stretches, covering a total distance of 1200 m. If, on the other hand, he runs repetitions of 100 m at the same speed, allowing intervals of 30 seconds between them, he will not incur any lactic acid production. In four hours he can perform 360 cycles covering a total 36 000 m. He will thus perform 30 times as much work as he could have done had the exercise been continuous (Margaria 1976).

At lower rates of power output, such as those required in long-distance running, the aerobic metabolism of glycogen, glucose, and fatty acids can provide the ATP necessary for contraction. Under these conditions, fatigue is likely to arise from a depletion of liver and muscle glycogen and free fatty acids derived from adipose tissue.

Muscle fibre type and fatigue

The response of a muscle fatigue will depend, in part, on the type of muscle fibres of which it is composed. Fast-twitch fibres tend to have higher levels of phosphocreatine and glycogen, than slow muscle. Gollnick, Karlsoon, Piehl, and Saltin (1974) have shown that in exercises involving near-maximal contractions, fast-twitch fibres are depleted of glycogen first, whereas at submaximal levels of exercise slow-twitch fibres are the first to be depleted of glycogen.

Summary and conclusions

In summary, it may be said that the site of fatigue in muscle depends on the intensity of exercise. At the very highest rate of exercise there will be a tendency towards intermittent failure of neuro-muscular transmission and muscle action potential accompanied by a rapid depletion of phosphocreatine and a rise in ADP which may lead to the observed failure of excitation–contraction coupling. At slightly lower work rates which can be continued for two to three minutes, there will be a substantial accumulation of lactate and hydrogen ions which probably also leads to failures of excitation-contraction coupling. At the lowest work rates, where the exercise can be continued for hours, fatigue is probably caused by depletion of liver and muscle glycogen.

References

Asmussen, E. and Mazin, B. (1978). A central nervous component in local muscular fatigue. *Eur. J. appl. Physiol.* **38**, 9–15.

Bigland-Ritchie, B., Jones, D. A., and Woods, J. J. (1979). Excitation frequency and muscle fatigue: electrical responses during human voluntary and stimulated contractions. *Exp. Neurol.* **64**, 414–27.

Dawson, M. J., Gadian, D. G., and Wilkie, D. R., (1978). Muscular fatigue investigated by phosphorus nuclear magnetic resonance. *Nature, Lond.* **273**, 861–6.

—— (1980). Mechanical relaxation rate and metabolism studied in fatiguing muscle by phosphorus nuclear magnetic resonance. *J. Physiol.* **299**, 461–84.

Edwards, R. H. T., Hill, D. K., and Jones, D. A., (1975). Metabolic changes associated with the slowing of relaxation in fatigued mouse muscle. *J. Physiol.* **251**, 287–301.

Gandevia, S. C. and McCloskey, D. I. (1977). Effects of related sensory inputs on motor performances in man studied through changes in perceived heaviness. *J. Physiol.* **272**, 653–72.

Gollnick, P. D., Karlsson, J., Piehl, K., and Saltin, B. (1974). Selective glycogen depletion in skeletal muscle fibres of man following sustained contraction. *J. Physiol.* **261**, 59–67.

Grabowski, W., Lobsiger, E. A., and Luttgau, H. C. (1972). The effect of repetitive stimulation at low frequencies upon the electrical and mechanical activity of single muscle fibres. *Pflügers Arch. ges. Physiol.* **334**, 222–39.

Harris, R. C., Edwards, R. H. T., Hultman, E., Nordesjo, L. O., Nylind, B. and Sahlin, K. (1976). The time course of phosphorylcreatine resynthesis during recovery of quadriceps muscle in man. *Pflügers Arch. ges. Physiol.* **367**, 137–42.

Ikai, M., Yabe, K., and Ischii, K. (1967). Muskelkraft und musculare erdmunding bie Willkurlicher anspanning und Electrischer Reizung des Muskels. *Sportsarzund Sportmedizn* **5**, 197–211.

Jones, D. A. (1979). Change in excitation threshold as a cause of muscular fatigue. *J. Physiol.* **295**, 90–1.

—— Bigland-Ritchie, B., and Edwards, R. H. T. (1979). Excitation frequency and muscle fatigue: mechanical responses during voluntary and stimulated contractions. *Exp. Neurol.* **64**, 401–13.

Krnjevic, K. and Miledi, R. (1958). Failure of neuromuscular propagation in rat. *J. Physiol.* **140**, 440–61.

Luttgau, H. C. (1965). The effect of metabolic inhibitors on the fatigue of the action potential in single muscle fibres. *J. Physiol.* **178**, 45–67.

Margaria, R. (1976). *Biomechanics and energetics of muscular exercise.* Clarendon Press, Oxford.

Marsden, C. D., Meadows, J. C., and Merton, P. A. (1976). Fatigue in human muscle in relation to the number and frequency of motor impulses. *J. Physiol.* **258**, 94P.

Newsholme, E. A. (1977). The regulation of intracellular and extracellular fuel supply during sustained exercise. The marathon: physiological, medical, epidemiological, and psychological studies. *Ann. N. Y. Acad. Sci.* **301**, 81–91.

Stephens, J. A., and Taylor, A. (1972). Fatigue of maintained voluntary contraction in man. *J. Physiol.* **220**, 1–18.

3 Factors affecting running performance

B. DAVIES AND P. JAKEMAN

Introduction

Of the many factors that influence running performance, maximal oxygen uptake ($\dot{V}O_2$ max), the ability to utilize a high percentage of $\dot{V}O_2$ max for sustained periods, muscle fibre composition, and muscle respiratory capacity, have been identified as the principal physiological determinants of the endurance athlete.

Maximal oxygen uptake is a reliable indicator of cardio-respiratory performance (Shephard, Allen, Benade, Davies, DiPrampero, Hedman, Merriman, Myhre, and Simmons 1968; Taylor, Buskirk, and Henschel 1955) and, as such, has been used as a criterion of endurance performance capacity (Costill 1967; Rusko, Havu, and Karvinen 1978; Wyndham, Strydom, Rensburg, and Benade 1969). The maximum oxygen consumption an athlete can attain is thought to be a product of genetic endowment and training (Pollock 1973), and the consistently high values recorded by elite runners suggest that a high $\dot{V}O_2$ max is an important prerequisite for success. Although $\dot{V}O_2$ max differentiates well in athletes of diverse abilities, there is a limitation of using $\dot{V}O_2$ max alone as a predictor of running performance in highly specialized groups of elite runners. Following several years of intensive endurance training, $\dot{V}O_2$ max has been shown to become a relatively stable feature of the athlete's physiological profile (Daniels 1974a), whilst running performances continue to improve. It would seem that improved performance in the endurance trained athlete may not be detected by change in $\dot{V}O_2$ max alone.

A significant relationship has been established between $\dot{V}O_2$ max and muscle respiratory capacity (Bergh, Thorstensson, Sjödin, Hulten, Piehl, and Karlsson 1978; Costill, Daniels, Evans, Fink, Krahenbuhl, and Saltin 1976; Foster, Costill, Daniels, and Fink 1978; Saltin, Henriksson, Nygaard, Anderson, and Johnson 1977) that is dependent on both muscle fibre composition and cross-sectional area (Essen, Jansson, Henriksson, Taylor, and Saltin 1975). With regard to muscle fibre composition, the relative distribution of slow twitch (ST) to fast twitch (FT) shows a marked predominance of ST fibres in the leg muscles of elite distance runners (Costill, Fink, and Pollock 1976; Gollnick, Armstrong, Saubert, Piehl, and Saltin 1972). These findings fit well with the metabolic characteristics of the fibres and the function they perform.

Longitudinal studies have shown that both the $\dot{V}O_2$ and oxidative potential of the muscle can be improved by training (Gollnick, Armstrong, Saltin, Saubert, Sembrowich, and Shepherd 1973) and that the augmentation of mitochondrial enzyme activity, capillary density, and enhancement of FFA oxidation is localized in the fibres most active in the training programme and has been shown to occur in both ST and FT fibre types (Henriksson and Reitman 1977b). Thus, low-intensity training gave rise to increases in ST oxidative capacity, whilst during high-intensity interval training the largest increase in succinic dehydrogenase (SDH) activity was found in the FT fibres. During the period over which the time of peak performance capacity can be attained, the level of adaptation is maximal (Henriksson and Reitman 1977a), resulting in a high rate of lipid oxidation and a lowered rate of glycogen utilization and lactate production. Both these metabolic factors are of primary importance for the observed enhanced work capacity.

Recently a measure has been introduced, originally termed the anaerobic threshold (An-T), that would more adequately describe the circulatory and metabolic adaptations that occur, and which could be used as a prediction measure of endurance performance which is dependent upon aerobic and anaerobic power (Wasserman, Whipp, Koyal, and Beaver 1973; Davis, Vodak, Wilmore, Vodak, and Kurtz 1976). As originally described, the An-T was defined to be the work rate of $\dot{V}O_2$ just below the onset of an anaerobiosis, as determined by the increase in blood lactate above resting levels during graded exercise (Leisen, Mader, Heck, and Hollman 1977). There is still conflict regarding the onset of anaerobiosis in man but it is now more generally agreed that the initial onset of lactate production that marks the upper limit of an exclusive aerobic metabolism (and is associated with several non–invasive measures, e.g. non-linear in $\dot{V}_E$ and $\dot{V}CO_2$), be termed the aerobic threshold, the anaerobic threshold being the work load or $\dot{V}O_2$ following an abrupt and continuous rise in lactate, with a mean concentration of lactate at this point of around 4 mM (Mader, Leisen, Heck, Philippi, Rost, Schurch, and Hollmann 1976).

The importance of this measure is probably reflected in the numerous publications that have recently appeared on the subject (e.g., MacDougall, 1977; Kindermann, Simon, and Keul 1979; Green, Daub, Painter, Houston, and Thomson 1979; Rusko, Rahkila, and Karvinen 1980), but none more so than the recent finding of a high positive correlation between muscle respiratory capacity and the lactate threshold and the percentage of ST fibres and the lactate threshold (Ivy, Withers, Handel, Elger, and Costill 1980). This, coupled with the evidence that the running speed related to the onset of plasma lactate is significantly correlated to performance and race pace in distance running (Farrell, Wilmore, Coyle, Billing, and Costill 1979), make it an important feature of the athlete's physiological profile.

It is well established that endurance is a function of relative work rate, i.e.

the greater the percentage of one's $\dot{V}O_2$ max required for the performance of the activity, the shorter the duration that it can be continued (Åstrand and Rodahl 1970). The ability to perform prolonged exercises at a high percentage of one's $\dot{V}O_2$ max is a further characteristic of the endurance performer (Costill, Thomason, and Roberts 1973), although a recent paper suggests that performance is more closely related to the ability to maintain a large absolute oxygen consumption, independent of what fraction of $\dot{V}O_2$ max this represents (Farrell *et al.* 1979). It has also been suggested that running economy, defined as the relationship between oxygen consumption and running speed, may also be related to performance (Daniels 1974b; Bransford and Howley 1977; Conley and Krahenbuhl 1980). Large inter-individual variation in running economy (Pollock 1977) in heterogeneous groups has been reported, but this factor has not been investigated by a longitudinal study as to the effects of training.

Experimental

In August 1978 we initiated a longitudinal study (15 months) to investigate the variation of $\dot{V}O_2$ max, anaerobic threshold, and running economy in a group of 16 highly trained middle-distance athletes (Table 3.1) during a full season of training and competitive athletics.

Table 3.1 *Physiological characteristics and running times for middle-distance athletes*

Subject	Age (y)	Weight (kg)	Height (cm)	Estimated % fat	$\dot{V}O_2$ max (ml kg/min)	Running times (min) 800m	1500m	3000m
MM	18	63.0	177.5	9.2	78.9	1.52	3.44	8.00
PB	17	64.9	177.1	9.0	76.1	1.50	3.52	8.16
CM	18	63.0	175.9	11.5	74.1	1.51	3.58	8.17
PL	19	70.2	178.2	12.2	71.2	1.52	3.49	8.22
KO	17	57.3	173.3	9.9	75.4	1.53	3.52	8.21
AS	18	60.3	180.2	12.9	81.1	1.57	3.57	8.45
DJ	17	59.4	170.1	15.0	75.2	1.56	3.57	8.31
JD	16	54.1	169.1	9.4	72.4	1.59	4.02	8.44
BS	19	72.2	183.6	15.5	79.5	2.03	4.07	8.37
PB	20	65.9	177.9	11.5	76.0	2.03	4.08	8.38
Mean	18	63.0	176.3	11.6	75.9	1.55	3.56	8.25
SD	±1.14	±5.2	±4.2	±2.2	±3.0	±4.3(s)	±7.4(s)	±13.8(s)
JP	20	60.1	175.6	23.5	65.2	2.03	4.20	
JW	19	47.6	163.1	17.2	68.6	2.08	4.14	
JL	20	53.9	170.9	18.4	70.6	1.04	4.14	
JC	16	50.9	160.2	22.5	63.0	2.07	4.24	
DR	16	55.8	168.9	20.5	64.2	2.17	4.44	
JK	16	52.4	165.9	19.9	65.6	2.18	4.43	
Mean	17.83	53.5	167.4	20.3	66.2	2.09	4.20	
SD	±1.86	±3.9	±5.1	±2.2	±2.6	±5.9(s)	±16.5(s)	

$\dot{V}o_2$ max was determined by a modification of the procedure described by Costill and Fox (1969). The test protocol required a warm-up period of five minutes at 12.5 kpH, after which a one-minute rest was given. After the warm-up the test began at an exercise pace of 17.5 kpH for males and 15.0 kpH for female athletes. At each successive two-minute interval the treadmill was raised by 2.5 per cent until exhaustion. Using this protocol all the subjects tested terminated the test within 6–10 minutes. The point of exhaustion, whilst variable amongst individual athletes, produced little intra-individual variation resulting in a test-retest correlation of 0.96 for 22 subjects (16 male and six female) retested within a three-day period.

Criteria for the attainment of $\dot{V}o_2$ max

Different investigators advocate different individual or multiple standards for determining when $\dot{V}o_2$ max has been reached. Within the present sensitivity of measurement it is accepted that maximum oxygen uptake has been reached when the oxygen response ($\dot{V}o_2$) is less than 150 ml (2 ml/kg/min) for two consecutive increases in work load, i.e. a 1–2 per cent increase in slope (Taylor, Haskell, Fox, and Blackburn 1969). Subsidiary criteria for a true maximum include physiological evidence of tissue hypoxia as reflected by (1) a respiratory exchange ratio of between 1.15–1.20 (Issekutz, Birkhead, and Rodahl 1962) and (2) an arterial lactate concentration > 8–9 mM (Åstrand and Rodahl 1970), in addition to a heart rate close to the age-predicted maximum (Shephard *et al.* 1968).

In highly trained athletes a normal $\dot{V}o_2$ plateau was not always evident and the respiratory exchange ratio did not always rise above 1.15, an observation also noted by Costill and Winrow (1970). However, comparatively high values, often > 14.0 mM lactate, were recorded suggesting a high level of anaerobic metabolism. Invariably all the athletes tested satisfied at least two of the following criteria.

(1) $\dot{V}o_2$ plateau equivalent to < 100 ml $\dot{V}o_2$ during the last two minutes of exercise.
(2) Blood lactate > 10 mM for male; > 8 mM for female athletes, with a post-exercise (+ 5 min) increase in lactate concentration.
(3) Heart rate attaining maximum during the last two minutes of exercise.

The recorded value for $\dot{V}o_2$ max was the highest value attained throughout the test.

$\dot{V}o_2$*-related running economy*

The aerobic requirement of submaximal treadmill running has been shown to be directly proportional to running speed (Margaria, Cerretelli, Aghemo, and Sassi 1963a,b; Pugh 1970) and has been calculated to be approximately 200 ml/kg/km. Data on running economy have been obtained by the measurement of the $\dot{V}O_2$ required for steady-state running at varying submaximal running speeds (Costill *et al.* 1973; Pollock 1977; Conley and Krahenbuhl 1980) and assumes that (a) treadmill running adequately reflects normal track running (McMiken and Daniels 1976) and (b) the measured $\dot{V}O_2$ represents the total energy required during submaximal work (Margaria *et al.* 1963b; Whipp, Seard, and Wasserman 1970).

For this study each subject completed six runs of six-minutes' duration at 228, 255, 282, 308, 335, and 363 m/min with 20 minutes recovery between each run. Expired gas was collected during the last two minutes of each run using a meteorological balloon and low resistance breathing valve (Jakeman and Davies 1978). The mean $\dot{V}O_2$ recorded for this two-minute period was taken as the aerobic requirement for each speed. The relationship between $\dot{V}O_2$ and running speed was described by the regression equation.

$$\dot{V}O_2 = \text{constant} \times \text{running speed} + \text{intercept (Fig. 3.1)}$$

Determination of the aerobic threshold

The determination of the aerobic threshold was based upon the work load or $\dot{V}O_2$ corresponding to an initial rise in plasma lactate above resting levels that occurs during a gradual incremental work test. Repeated blood samples for blood lactate were taken initially from finger-prick samples and finally from

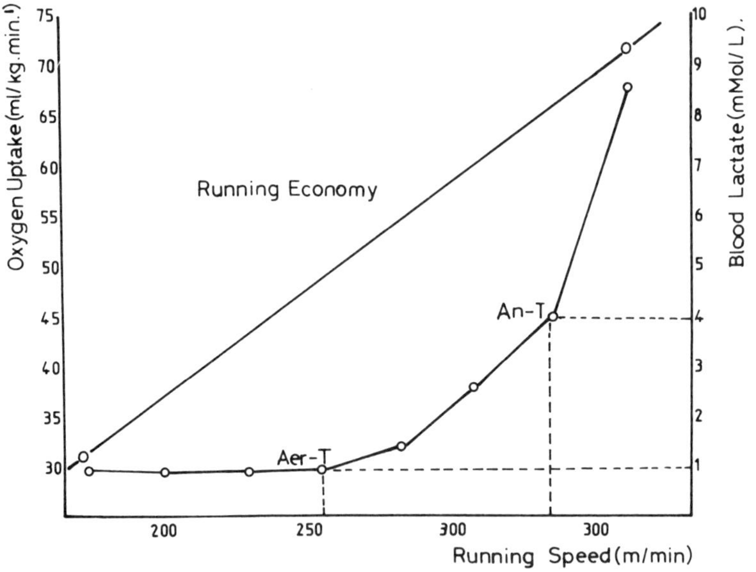

Fig. 3.1. A relationship between maximal aerobic power, running economy, and the anaerobic threshold.

a 19 gauge indwelling catheter for the test proper. During the latter part of the work the aerobic threshold was also assessed from respiratory gas-exchange indices as described by Wasserman *et al.* (1973). Respiratory gas-exchange parameters were monitored at 30-second intervals throughout the test, with the aid of a Beckman Metabolic Measurement Cart (MMC). Several protocols were evaluated and the aerobic threshold obtained from the lactate values was compared with that obtained when a line of best fit was drawn through the points of abrupt change in $\dot{V}_E$, $\dot{V}_{CO_2}$, and FE_{CO_2} as described by Davis *et al.* (1976). Caution should be exercised when determination of the aerobic threshold is made from respiratory gas-exchange indices alone. Initial evaluation of this procedure yielded aerobic threshold estimates within ±30 seconds of those determined from lactate values. This work, undertaken with non-endurance trained subjects, required individual adjustment of the magnitude of the work load required for each subject in order to produce a satisfactory response. Estimates of the aerobic threshold with highly trained endurance athletes based solely upon respiratory gas-exchange parameters often produced several possible criteria, making the determination of the aerobic threshold tentative.

Determination of the anaerobic threshold

Determination of the anaerobic threshold was based upon the direct measurement of lactic acid (Leisen *et al.* 1977; Mader *et al.* 1976; Mader, Heck, and Hollmann 1978). The anaerobic threshold was defined as the work load or $\dot{V}_{O_2}$ that was followed by an abrupt and continuous rise in lactic acid, with a mean concentration of lactate of 4 mM at this point. Because of the possible delay in the diffusion of lactate produced in the muscle entering the circulation and the initial rise in lactate at the onset of work, Mader and Hollmann (1977) suggested that the duration of the work load should be not less than four minutes, preferably longer.

In this study of treadmill running the observed abrupt and continuous rise in lactate approximated well with a lactate concentration of 4 mM. As there was a limit to the number of runs that could be undertaken in order to determine the exact point of increase in lactate, the $\dot{V}_{O_2}$ and running speed corresponding to the anaerobic threshold was determined by direct interpolation at the point of 4mM lactate (Fig. 3.1). This assessment was made from the six submaximal runs described previously in the section which deals with $\dot{V}_{O_2}$-related running economy.

Results and discussion

The physiological profile produced for each athlete (Fig. 3.1) illustrates the relationship between $\dot{V}_{O_2\,max}$ anaerobic threshold, and running economy. Figure 3.2 highlights some of the inter-individual differences that exist

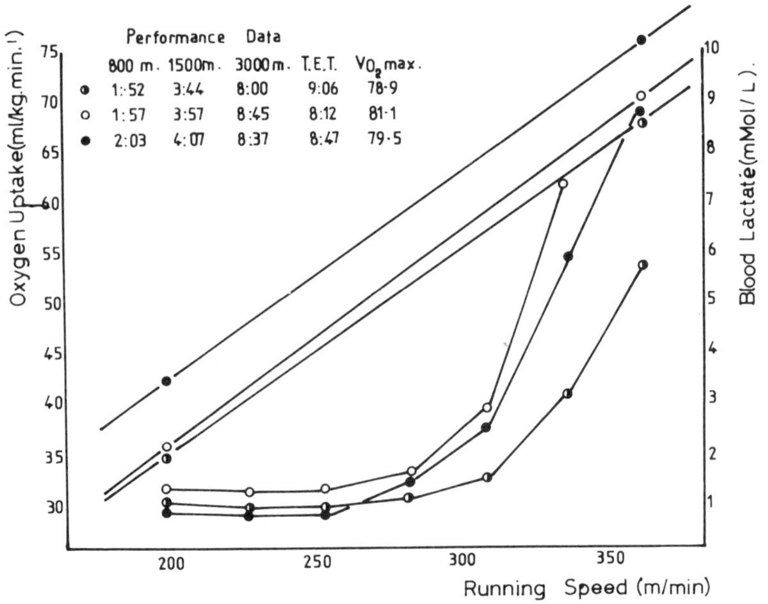

Fig. 3.2. Inter-individual differences in $\dot{V}O_2$ max, running economy, anaerobic threshold, and running times within the middle-distance group of athletes.

within the group. Although the three athletes illustrated possess approximately equivalent values for $\dot{V}O_2$ max there are substantial differences in performance, running economy, and the speed related to the anaerobic threshold (An-T).

The group was re-assessed on four occasions, post-season (September 1978), mid-winter (January 1979), pre-season (May 1979), and post-season (September 1979), the training undertaken throughout this period being consistent throughout the group (Table 3.2). The mean data for each of these testing session (Table 3.3) reveal a slight trend towards increases in the speed-related An-T and treadmill endurance times in the period leading to the start of the track season, although the overall change within the group was not significant. However, the overall results mask the intra-individual change observed for some of the subjects within the group. An example of this is given in Fig. 3.3 in which the increase in performance times for the selected events is reflected in both a positive increase in the running speed related to the anaerobic threshold and a significant change in running economy as described by the regression equation of $\dot{V}O_2$ upon running speed. No change in $\dot{V}O_2$ max was observed. A similar, but not always such a pronounced effect, was observed in four other athletes who had attained significant increases in performance times during the period of study.

If, as is suggested above, change in performance is partially reflected by

Table 3.2 *Summary of training programme undertaken during the period September 1978–September 1979*

Sept.–Oct. 1978	F	35–40 miles/week*	
	M	50 miles/week†	
Nov. 1978	F	35–40 miles/week	1 session per week, 4 × 1200 m
	M	50 miles/week	work : rest, 1 : 1
Dec. 1978	F	35–40 miles/week	2 sessions per week, 4 × 1200 m
	M	50 miles/week	work : rest, 1 : 1
Jan.–Feb. 1979	F	35 miles/week	1 session per week, 4 × 1200 m
	M	50 miles/week	1 session per week, 12 × 450 m
Feb.–Apr. 1979	F	35 miles/week	1 session per week 4 × 1200 m
	M	50 miles/week	1 session per week 200–300 m repeats
Apr.–Aug. 1979	F	Selected peaking schedules	
	M	for each individual athlete	
		prior to competition	

* Female athletes, 5-mile sessions at approx. 6-min 20-s pace.
† Male athletes, 5-mile sessions at approx. 5-min 40-s pace.

Table 3.3 *Mean change (ISD) in the physiological data of middle-distance athletes over the 12-month period of study*

	Post-season, Sept. 1978		Mid-winter, Dec. 1978		Pre-season, May 1979		Post-season, Sept. 1979	
Parameter	M	F	M	F	M	F	M	F
Max. aerobic power ($\dot{V}O_{2max}$ ml min)	5016 ±516	3428 ±387	4997 ±399	3499 ±374	5082 ±417	3541 ±341	4923 ±488	3477 ±291
Max. aerobic power ($\dot{V}O_{2max}$ (ml kg)/min)	75.7 ±2.3	63.4 ±2.2	76.8 ±3.2	63.6 ±1.4	75.8 ±3.17	62.8 ±1.2	73.4 ±3.04	61.8 ±2.0
Treadmill endurance time (min)	8.22 ±0.39	7.46 ±0.6	8.73 ±0.53	7.7 ±0.72	8.57 ±0.41	8.1 ±0.6	8.36 ±0.38	7.9 ±0.74
Anaerobic threshold speed (m min)	309 ±12	260 ±8.6	318.9 ±7.8	275 ±10.5	317 ±8.8	280 ±8.92	314 ±12	279 ±5.2
Aerobic threshold ($\dot{V}O_2$ max, (ml kg)/min)	62.2 ±3.8	52.7 ±2.6	63.5 ±4.2	55.9 ±3.6	65.0 ±3.1	54.2 ±4.0	61.5 ±4.1	53.6 ±2.74
Anaerobic threshold ($\dot{V}O_2$ % of max.)	81.9 ±5.9	82.8 ±6.01	83.8 ±5.3	88.5 ±6.4	85.8 ±4.3	87.0 ±6.8	84.3 ±6.2	86.5 ±2.0
($\dot{V}O_2$ at 268 m min ((ml kg)/min)	51.4 ±3.05	53.8 ±5.03	50.8 ±3.4	54.7 ±4.81	52.8 ±2.95	52.2 ±3.89	50.5 ±3.22	50.0 ±3.48

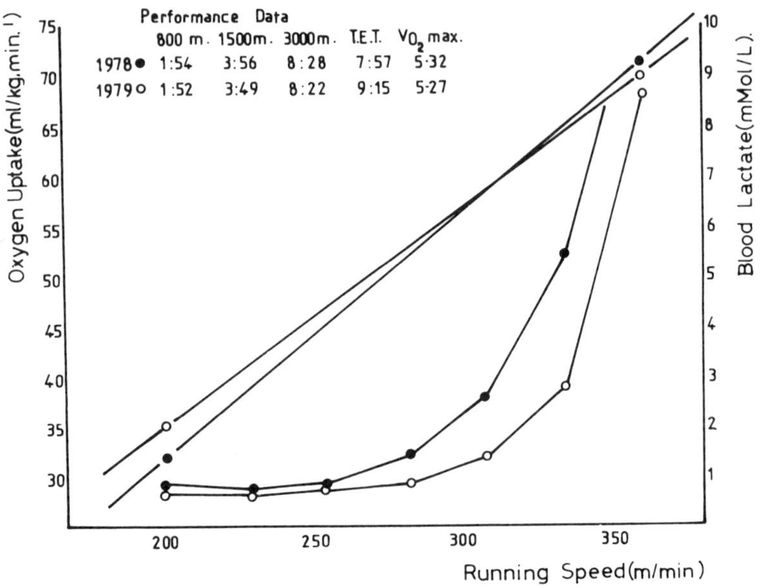

Fig. 3.3. An example of the intra-individual change in $\dot{V}O_{2\ max}$, running economy, anaerobic threshold, and performance times observed during the period of study.

change in the work load or $\dot{V}O_2$ associated with the anaerobic threshold, we thought it valuable to investigate the influence of differing training programmes upon the anaerobic threshold. Furthermore, it has been suggested that endurance training, when performed at an intensity below the anaerobic threshold, would only maintain the state of conditioning, for whilst leading to improvements in the cardio-vascular system the stimulus is not sufficient to achieve adequate adaptation in the muscle cells, whereas that performed in the region of the anaerobic threshold would enhance exercise capacity (Kindermann *et al.* 1979).

To test such an hypothesis, we trained two groups of subjects at an exercise intensity requiring one group to work above, and one below, the anaerobic threshold while maintaining the same physiological stimulus in terms of oxygen, i.e. subject A training below the An-T would train at an exercise intensity of 60 per cent $\dot{V}O_{2\ max}$ for 60 minutes, whilst subject B training above the An-T would train at an exercise intensity of 80 per cent $\dot{V}O_{2\ max}$ for 45 minutes. Each subject trained for periods ranging from 42 to 78 minuted per day, five days per week for eight weeks on a cycle ergometer. The subjects were assessed pre-, mid-, and post-training by a three-minute graded increment test similar to that described by Wasserman *et al.* (1973) and were randomly assigned their training loads either above or below the An-T. Throughout the period of training, pin-prick blood samples were

Table 3.4 *Mean change (and range) in aerobic and anaerobic thresholds with training*

			$\dot{V}O_2$-related aer-T		$\dot{V}O_2$-related an-T	
	$\dot{V}O_2$ max	Load max	Absolute	Relative	Absolute	Relative
Overall	+7.4% (2.3–17.8)	+19.9% (7.1–28.0)	+9.9%	+6.8%	+11.3%	+6.5%
Above An-T	+4.5% (2.3–8.2)	+16.9% (7.1–22.2)	+6.5%	+5.5%	+10.7%	+7.8%
Below An-T	+11.2% (5.3–17.8)	+23.5%	+13.6%	+7.5%	+11.9%	+4.3%

taken in order to confirm the training intensity. Plasma lactates at the end of the training period were 5.1 ±1.1 mM and 2.9 ±1.5 mM, respectively, for the two groups training above and below the An-T.

The overall change in $\dot{V}O_2$ max (Table 3.4) for both groups was 7.4 per cent, but the range was large (2.3–17.8 per cent). However, a significantly larger increase in $\dot{V}O_2$ max (11.2 *v*. 4.5 per cent) occurred in the group training below the An-T. Submaximally, this difference was reflected in a significantly greater increase in the $\dot{V}O_2$-related Aer-T (13.6 *v*.6.5 per cent) but no significant difference in the $\dot{V}O_2$-related An-T (11.9 *v*.10.7 per cent). In a similar study (Davis, Whipp, and Wasserman 1979) relating the effects of training on the Aer-T, a 16 per cent increase in Aer-T has been shown which was greater than, and independent of, a 7 per cent rise of $\dot{V}O_2$ max, whereas a 44 per cent rise in absolute Aer-T (15 per cent increase in relative terms) has been reported in a training study that produced a mean rise of 25 per cent in $\dot{V}O_2$ max (Williams, Wyndham, Kok, and Rahden 1967). The difference between the results is probably a reflection of the differing training methods and the initial fitness status of the subjects used.

The absolute change in An-T between the groups was very similar (11.9 *v*.10.7 per cent), but the relative change showed a larger increase in the group training above the An-T (7.8 *v*.4.3 per cent), although this difference was not significant. There is, to the authors' knowledge, no data to support this evidence in the literature.

The above data would suggest that the two training programmes, one above and one below the An-T (but requiring the same energy cost in terms of $\dot{V}O_2$), will produce differing cardio-respiratory and metabolic adaptations. Training below the An-T provides for greater enhancement of cardiovascular change coupled to a larger positive shift in the Aer-T that probably reflects a large increase in the oxidative capacity of the muscle cell. Training above the An-T, whilst not producing such a large increase in $\dot{V}O_2$ max, produced a relatively larger increase in the $\dot{V}O_2$-related An-T that possibly suggests a greater control of the glycolytic potential of the cell and/or increased inter-cellular metabolism of lactate, delaying the onset of a large increase in lactate into the bloodstream.

The elevation of the anaerobic threshold to a higher percentage of $\dot{V}O_{2\,max}$ would, in effect, produce a sparing effect upon muscle glycogen and thus increase the capacity of the subject to maintain a work load requiring a higher percentage of $\dot{V}O_{2\,max}$ for a sustained period of time.

A glycogen-sparing effect can also be produced by increasing the contribution of FFA oxidation to the total energy production of the muscle (Costill, Coyle, Dalsky, Evans, and Fink 1977). A recent study by Ivy, Costill, Fink, and Lower (1979) reported that elevation of FFA metabolism by ingestion of caffeine could increase endurance performance time by an average of 7 per cent. Preliminary data from this laboratory have shown that the effect of caffeine feeding will produce little change in the aerobic threshold but will elevate the $\dot{V}O_2$-related anaerobic threshold about 5 per cent. These preliminary findings may account for the enhanced work capacity produced by the elevation of FFA metabolism upon caffeine ingestion.

We have discussed several important physiological characteristics that could possibly influence athletic performance. Whilst recognizing the importance of a high aerobic capacity ($\dot{V}O_{2max}$) for endurance running, we also realize that other factors may be equally important for success at international level.

The terminology describing the inflection point of blood lactic acid concentration seems to be a very confusing issue. We recognize that this inflection point is influenced by training and is implicated in performance. However, physiological conclusions regarding muscle metabolism derived from blood lactate concentrations should be considered with caution. The lactic-acid inflection point represents an interaction between tissue metabolism, blood flow, entry rate, fractional removal, and production. Therefore, to equate the rapid increase in blood lactate concentration solely to muscle production would be misleading and unwise.

There is a substantial amount of variation in the running economy of heterogeneous groups, but it is quite possible that in a homogeneous group of highly trained athletes running economy may prove to be highly influential in competitive long-distance running.

Acknowledgements

The authors acknowledge the financial support of the Provincial Insurance Company and the assistance of the members of the Metabolic Profile Unit, University of Salford.

References

Åstrand, P. O. and Rodahl, K. (1970). *Textbook of work physiology*, pp. 291–3. McGraw-Hill, New York.

Bergh, U., Thorstensson, A., Sjödin, B., Hulten, B., Piehl, K., and Karlsson, J. (1978). Maximal oxygen uptake and muscle fibre types in trained and untrained humans. *Med. Sci. Sports* **10**, 151–4.

Bransford, D. R. and Howley, E. T. (1977). Oxygen cost of running in trained and untrained men and women. *Med. Sci. Sports* **9**, 41–4.

Conley, D. L. and Krahenbuhl, G. S. (1980). Running economy and distance running performance of highly trained athletes. *Med. Sci. Sports* **12**, 357–60.

Costill, D. L. (1967). The relationship between selected physiological variables and distance running performance. *J. Sports Med.* **7**, 61–6.

—— and Fox, E. L. (1969). Energetics of marathon running. *Med. Sci. Sports* **1**, 81–6.

—— and Winrow, E. (1970). Maximal oxygen intake among marathon runners. *Arch Phys. Med. Rehab.* **51**, 317–20.

—— Fink, J. W., and Pollock, M. L. (1976). Muscle fibre composition and enzyme activities of elite distance runners. *Med. Sci. Sports* **8**, 96–100.

—— Thomason, H. and Roberts, E. (1973). Fractional utilization of the aerobic capacity during distance running. *Med. Sci. Sports* **5**, 248–52.

—— Coyle, E., Dalsky, G., Evans, W., and Fink, J. W. (1977). Effects of elevated FFA and insulin on muscle glycogen usage during exercise. *J. appl. Physiol.* **43**, 695–99.

—— Daniels, J. T., Evans, W., Fink, J. W., Krahenbuhl, G. S., and Saltin, B. (1976). Skeletal muscle enzymes and fibre composition in male and female track athletes. *J. appl. Physiol.* **40**, 149–54.

Daniels, J. T. (1974a). Running with Jim Ryun: A five year study. *Phys. Sports Med.* **2**, 63–7.

—— (1974b). Physiological characteristics of champion male athletes. *Res. Quant.* **45**, 342–8.

Davis, J. A., Whipp, F. M., and Wasserman, K. (1979). Anaerobic threshold alterations consequent to endurance training in middle-aged men. *Med. Sci. Sports* **11**, 96–9.

—— Vodak, P., Wilmore, J. H., Vodak, J., and Kurtz, P. (1976). Anaerobic threshold and maximal aerobic power for three modes of exercise. *J. appl. Physiol.* **41**, 544–50.

Essen, B., Jansson, E., Henriksson, J., Taylor, A. W., and Saltin, B. (1975). Metabolic characteristics of fibre types in human skeletal muscle. *Acta physiol. scand.* **95**, 153–65.

Farrell, P. A., Wilmore, J. H., Coyle, E. F., Billing, J. E., and Costill, D. L. (1979). Plasma lactate accumulation and distance running performance. *Med. Sci. Sports* **11**, 338–44.

Foster, C., Costill, D. L ., Daniels, J. T., and Fink, J. W. (1978). Skeletal muscle enzyme activity, fibre composition and $\dot{V}O_{2\ max}$ in relation to distance running performance. *Eur. J. appl. Physiol.* **39**, 73–80.

Gollnick, P. D., Armstrong, R. B., Saubert, C. W. IV, Piehl, K., and Saltin, B. (1972). Enzyme activity and fibre composition in skeletal muscle of trained and untrained men. *J. appl. Physiol.* **33**, 312–19.

—— —— Saltin, B., Saubert, C. W. IV, Sembrowich, W. L., and Shepherd, R. E. (1973). Effect of training on enzyme activity and fibre composition in human skeletal muscle. *J. appl. Physiol.* **34**, 107–11.

Green, J., Daub, B., Painter, D., Houston, M., and Thomson, J. (1979). Anaerobic threshold and muscle fibre type, area and oxidative enzyme activity during graded cycling. *Med. Sci. Sports* **11**, 113–14.

Henriksson, J. and Reitman, J. S. (1977a). Time course activity changes in human skeletal muscle, SDH and cytochrome oxidase activities and maximal oxygen uptake in physical activity and inactivity. *Acta physiol. scand.* **99**, 91–7.

—— —— (1977b). Quantitative measures of enzyme activities in type I and type II muscle fibres in man after training. *Acts physiol. scand.* **97**, 392–7.

Issekutz, B., Birkhead, N. C., and Rodahl, H. (1962). Use of respiratory quotients in assessment of aerobic work capacity. *J. appl. Physiol.* **17**, 47–50.

Ivy, J. L., Costill, D. L., Fink, W. J., and Lower, R. W. (1979). Influence of caffeine and carbohydrate feedings on endurance performance. *Med. Sci. Sports* **11** 6–11.

—— Withers, R. T., Handel, P. J. van Elger, D. H., and Costill, D. L. (1980). Muscle respiratory capacity and fibre type as determinants of the lactate threshold. *J. appl. Physiol: Respirat. Environ. Exercise Physiol.* **48**, 523–7.

Jakeman, P. and Davies, B. (1978). The characteristics of a low resistance breathing valve designed for the measurement of high aerobic power. *Br. J. Sports Med.* **13**, 81–3.

Kindermann, W., Simon, G., and Keul, J. (1979). The significance of the aerobic-anaerobic transition for the determination of work load intensities during endurance training. *Eur. J. appl. Physiol.* **42**, 25–34.

Leisen, H., Mader, A., Heck, H., and Hollmann, W. (1977). Die ausdauerleistungsfahigkeit bei verscheidenen sportarten under besonderer berucksichtigung des metabolismus: Zur ermittlung der optimalen belastungsintensitat im training. *Leistungssport* **9**, 63–79.

MacDougall, J. D. (1977). The anaerobic threshold: its significance for the endurance athlete. *Can. J. appl. Sports. Sci.* **2**, 137–40.

McMiken, D. F. and Daniels, J. T. (1976). Aerobic requirements and maximum aerobic power in treadmill and track running. *Med. Sci. Sports* **8**, 14–17.

Mader, A. and Hollmann, W. (1977). Zur bedeutung der stoffwechselleistungsfahigkeit des eliteruderers im training under wettkampf. *Leistungssport* **9**, 8–62.

—— Heck, H., and Hollmann, W. (1978). Evaluation of lactic acid anaerobic energy contribution by determination of post exercise lactic acid concentration of ear lobe capillary blood in middle-distance runners and swimmers. In *The International congress of physical activity sciences* (eds. F. Landry and W. Orban) Vol. 4. Symposia Specialists, Miami.

—— Leisen, H., Heck, H., Philippi, H., Rost, R., Schurch, P., and Hollmann, W. (1976). Zur beurteilung der sportartspezifischen ausdauerleistungs-fahigkeit im labor. *Sportarzt und Sportmedizin.* **27**, 80–8.

Margaria, R. P., Cerretelli, P., Aghemo, P., and Sassi, G. (1963a). The energy cost of running. *J. appl. Physiol.* **18**, 367–70.

—— —— DiPrampero, P. E., Massari, C., and Torelli, G. (1963b). Kinetics and mechanism of oxygen debt contraction in man. *J. appl. Physiol.* **18**, 371–7.

Pollock, M. L. (1973). The quantification of endurance training programs. In *Exercise and sports science reviews* (ed. J. H. Wilmore) Vol. 1. Academic Press, New York.

—— (1977). Submaximal and maximal working capacity of elite distance runners. Part 1: Cardiorespiratory aspects. *Ann. N.Y. Acad. Sci.* **301**, 310–22.

Pugh, L. G. C. E. (1970). Oxygen intake in track and treadmill running with observations on the effect of air resistance. *J. Physiol (Lond.)* **207**, 823–35.

Rusko, H., Havu, M., and Karvinen, E. (1978). Aerobic performance capacity in athletes. *Eur. J. appl. Physiol.* **38**, 151–9.
—— Rahkila, P., and Karvinen, E. (1980). Anaerobic threshold, skeletal muscle enzymes and fibre composition in young female cross-country skiers. *Acta physiol. scand.* **108**, 263–8.
Saltin, B., Henriksson, J., Nygaard, E., Anderson, P., and Johnson, E. (1977). Fibre types and metabolic potentials of skeletal muscles in sedentary man and endurance runners. *Ann. N. Y. Acad. Sci.* **301**, 3–29.
Shephard, R. J., Allen, C., Benade, A. J. S., Davies, C. T. M., DiPrampero, P. E., Hedman, R., Merriman, J. E., Myhre, K., and Simmons, R. (1968). The maximal oxygen intake – an international reference standard of cardiorespiratory fitness. *Bull. Wld Hlth Org.* **38**, 757–64.
Taylor, H. L., Buskirk, E., and Henschel, A. (1955). Maximal oxygen intake as an objective measure of cardiorespiratory performance. *J. appl. Physiol.* **8**, 73–80.
—— Haskell, W. L., Fox, S. M., and Blackburn, H. (1969). Exercise tests: A summary of procedures and concepts of stress testing for cardiovascular diagnosis and function evaluation. In *Measurement in exercise electrocardiography* (ed. H. Blackburn). Thomas, Springfield, Iu.
Wasserman, K., Whipp, B. J., Koyal, S. N., and Beaver, W. L. (1973). Anaerobic threshold and respiratory gas exchange during exercise. *J. appl Physiol.* **35**, 236–43.
Whipp, B. J., Seard, C., and Wasserman, K. (1970). Oxygen deficit – oxygen debt relationship and efficiency of anaerobic work. *J. appl. Physiol.* **23**, 452–6.
Williams, C. G., Wyndham, C. H., Kok, R., and Rahden, M. von (1967). Effects of training on maximum oxygen consumption and on anaerobic metabolism in man. *Int. angelw. Physiol.* **24**, 18–23.
Wyndham, C. H., Strydom, N. B., Rensburg, A. Y. van, and Benade, A. J. S. (1969). Physiological requirements for world class performances in endurance running. *S. Afr. Med. J.* **43**, 996–1002.

4 Performance and blood reinfusion

B. EKBLOM

'Blood doping' became of world-wide interest during the 1976 Olympic Games in Montreal. One of the greatest athletes in these games, Lasse Virén of Finland, was accused by the media of having been 'blood doped', as he was unwise enough to win two gold medals (5000 and 10 000 m) in Montreal, as he had done in Munich four years earlier. Because, in the years between these two Games, he had been a rather average performer, his remarkable performances on these occasions were regarded by his antagonists as resulting from 'blood doping'.

The question as to whether Virén really was 'blood doped' is of rather limited interest because, by looking at his performance and his training background, it has been suggested that his results can be explained by other means. However, this affair focused physiological interest on the effects of manipulation of haemoglobin concentration and blood volume on physical performance and circulation.

The background for this commenced in 1962, when I started experiments on the effects of physical training on central circulation and related physiological variables. As is well known, total haemoglobin as well as blood volume increases with training, and one of the questions that arose from these first experiments was how physical performance, maximal aerobic power, and central haemodynamics would be altered if the oxygen-carrying capacity of the blood is increased or decreased, and if the blood volume is acutely changed.

Knowing that some groups had already done some minor experiments (Gullbring, Holmgren, Sjöstrand, and Strandell 1960; Rowell 1962; Robinson, Epstein, Kahler, and Braunwald 1966), we started our work in 1966 and, after changes in the design of the experiments, our first results were published in 1970. Following some newspaper reports at around that time, the results of these experiments and the consequences for sport became a matter of some interest in Sweden. In 1971 *Track and Field News* in the United States included a short article about this, but it was not until 1976 that the work became of interest to a larger public. By the end of 1970, as a consequence of our experiments, several groups were investigating the effects of blood doping on different physiological parameters, e.g. Williams, Goodwin, Perkins, and Bocrie 1973; Buick, Gledhill, Froese, Spriet, and Meyers 1980).

Before referring to these experiments in detail, let us consider some basic exercise physiology and indicate our approach to the manipulation of the different links in the oxygen-transport-system chain and its consequences for maximal aerobic power, physical performance, and so on.

Physical performance, in general, can be determined by three main factors, namely, energy liberation, neuromuscular function, and physiological factors. The relative importance of each factor varies with the type of physical performance. In the following we have been mainly concerned with running uphill on a treadmill and bicycling. In these cases maximum aerobic power ($\dot{V}O_{2\ max}$) is considered to be a very important determinant of physical performance. We used standardized tests, i.e. individual speed and slope on the treadmill, and by 'physical performance' we mean time to exhaustion under these standard conditions. Thus, if we change one factor within the oxygen-transport-system chain, this change may alter maximal aerobic power, keeping other factors unchanged, and this may induce changes in physical performance. Whether this is a good way of measuring performance is a matter for discussion, but 20 years of experience with such tests suggests that this way of describing changes in physical performance is useful provided that it is used carefully.

What sets the limit to maximal aerobic power? Experiments carried out on the different muscle groups involved (Bergh, Kanstrup, and Ekblom 1976) indicates that although muscle mass may influence oxygen uptake during maximal exercise – as in separate arm work – the muscle mass does not set the upper limit for maximal aerobic power. This means that the central circulation is somehow involved, and it was against this background that experiments with the manipulation of different links in the oxygen-transport-system chain and corresponding consequence for circulation during exercise were undertaken.

The main experiments in this field have been concerned with the increase and decrease of haemoglobin concentration. Initially, the effects of repeated withdrawals of 400 ml of whole blood were studied. Maximal aerobic power was reduced in small steps, as was physical performance (Ekblom, Goldbarg, and Gullbring 1972).

The next stage involved the withdrawal of 800 ml of blood. Three well-trained physical education students were tested several times before blood withdrawal; after blood withdrawal they were studied several times at regular intervals until 27 days after the start of the experiment. The red cells (about 400 ml) were then reinfused. The blood had been stored in a blood bank in an adenin-ADC-solution. It was hypothesized that the athletes' haemoglobin concentrations would have returned to the original levels after 27 days and following reinfusion of the blood cells the haemoglobin concentration would be increased. After the reinfusion the subjects were again studied under the standardized conditions of slope and speed on the treadmill.

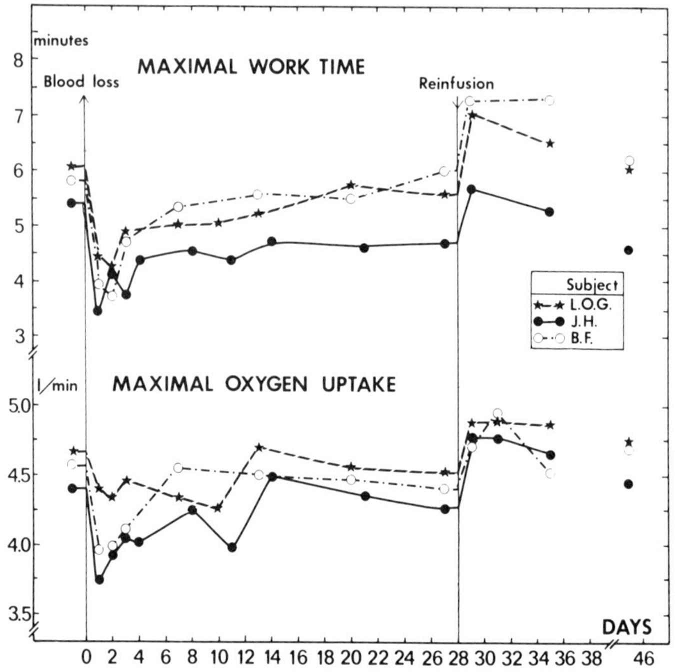

Fig. 4.1. The effects of blood withdrawal and subsequent reinfusion on maximal work times and maximal oxygen uptake.

The results of these experiments are shown in Fig. 4.1, and have given rise to discussion on several points:

(1) The 'placebo effect'. In my opinion, unless there has been some serious mistake in methodology, there is no way in which maximal aerobic power could be increased or decreased so rapidly 'overnight' as it did between days 27 and 28. This 'objection' must be regarded as non-physiological and of limited importance. With regard to 'physical performance' it is obvious that there are no clearly defined end-points in laboratory maximal tests of the kind adopted. A subject can almost always extend his work time by a few seconds more. The only recourse is to urge subjects to do their best on all tests and to give them maximum encouragement. Afterwards, data on blood lactate, heart rate, ventilation, etc., can be compared with those obtained before blood withdrawal and reinfusion, respectively. In the case of our work, blood lactate was lower after bleeding than before, which can be explained partly by the reduced work time. However, after reinfusion blood lactate was also somewhat lower than before, which confirms that the data on maximal aerobic power are not overestimated.

Pulmonary ventilation was unchanged throughout the experiment, as was the subjective rating of perceived exertion, as evaluated through the Borg scale. There are no reasons to believe that a subjective bias could explain the 'overnight' increase in maximal aerobic power, but on the other hand, psychological factors may have modified the magnitude of the changes in 'physical performance' as evaluated from time to exhaustion on the standardized maximal exercise. There are also no reasons to believe that, as has been suggested, the test between bleeding and reinfusion would generate a training effect, so that this would show up 'overnight' in parallel with the reinfusion of red blood cells.

(2) A second possible criticism lies within basic physiology. An increased haemoglobin concentration would theoretically increase viscosity. In earlier studies we have shown that many extremely well-trained athletes have a fairly low haemoglobin concentration at rest and, furthermore, the haemoconcentration from rest to maximal exercise in these athletes is fairly small, compared to non-athletes (Ekblom and Hermansen 1968). This argues against a positive effect of reinfusion on maximal aerobic power. However, direct measurements of cardiac output during maximal exercise do not support this as maximal cardiac output appears about the same in all the three experimental situations (Ekblom, Wilson, and Åstrand 1976).

(3) Another objection has been that the blood affinity to oxygen was changed during the weeks in the blood bank. Measurements of the 2.3-DPG at rest and during submaximal and maximal exercise showed an unchanged level in all the three experimental situations (Ekblom *et al.* 1976).

In my view, therefore, although one can criticize this study on the grounds that there was no control group with which to evaluate an eventual 'bias' from blood loss and reinfusion on 'performance', it is obvious that the increased maximal aerobic power can only be explained by the reinfusion of the red blood cells. Evidently, the peripheral working muscles are able to use this increased amount of available oxygen; this has been questioned, but our data, as well as studies from other laboratories (Buick *et al.* 1980; Spriet, Gledhill, Froese, Wilkes, and Meyers 1980), do not support such an objection.

These studies raised both physiological and 'practical' questions, some of which will be discussed below. As shown in Fig. 4.1 maximal aerobic power returned to prebleeding level after 14 days, despite the fact that haemoglobin concentration was still much reduced. At this point blood volume was increased. Thus, it seemed that an increased blood volume – at least in part – compensated for the decreased haemoglobin concentration. In order to study this particular question a further series of experiments was performed in which blood volume and haemoglobin concentration were altered independently of each other. In the first set of experiments, we increased blood volume with a plasma expander (Macrode®). The results are shown in Fig. 4.2.

It was a considerable surprise to note that $\dot{V}_{O_2 \, max}$ was not changed despite

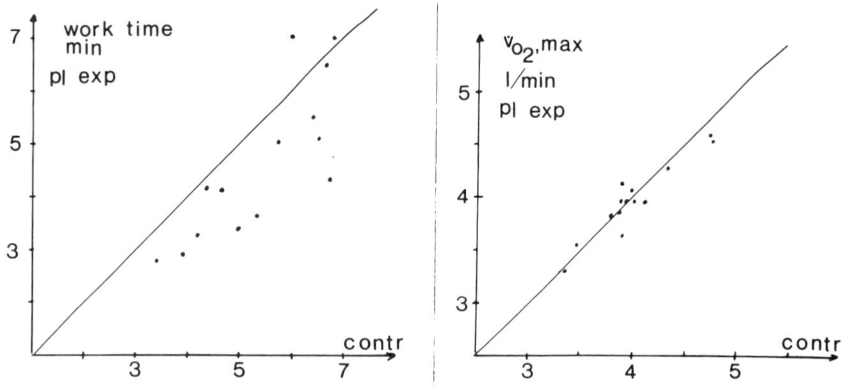

Fig. 4.2. The effects of plasma expansion on work time and maximal oxygen consumption.

a reduction in haemoglobin concentration during maximal exercise from an average 158 to 145 g/l. Physical performance was reduced as indicated in the upper part of Fig. 4.2. When the subjects were subjected to blood loss, reducing haemoglobin concentration by an equal amount, maximal aerobic power and physical performance were reduced, as shown in earlier studies (i.e. Ekblom *et al.* 1972, 1976).

Since blood-volume expansion evidently affected circulation, both at rest and during exercise up to maximum, it was decided to measure cardiac output in some subjects. At rest and during exercise, cardiac output was increased above corresponding data. Figure 4.3 shows data from maximal exercise. It is shown that stroke volume is markedly increased while heart rate is somewhat depressed, giving an increased cardiac output during maximal exercise. In this situation, central circulation can evidently adjust itself and at least partly compensate for the reduced haemoglobin concentration, when the blood volume is increased, but not when the blood volume is 'normal'.

What of the 'non-physiological' consequences of our research? It should be emphasized that these experiments were not performed in order to manipulate athletes or for some other such reasons.

Does manipulation of this kind really increase performance in sports events? In the early 1970s the results of studies of this question were published. A few of them did not show any positive effects of infusions of red blood cells, but some very serious mistakes occurred in these studies (i.e. Williams *et al.* 1972). For example, only 400 ml of blood was withdrawn and in one study the blood was reinfused some 14–17 days later. Haemoglobin concentration was not measured at all. These are serious criticisms since we have done some 30–35 experiments with reinfusion during the last 8–10 years and in four or five cases there was no increase in haemoglobin concen-

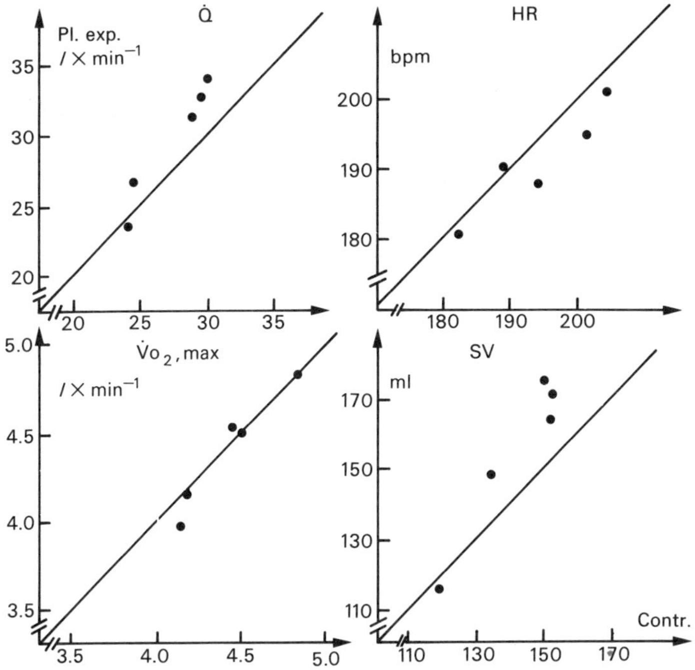

Fig. 4.3. The effects of plasma expansion on cardiac output ($\dot{Q}$) heart rate (HR) maximal oxygen consumption ($\dot{V}O_{2\ max}$), and stroke volume (SV) during maximal exercise.

tration after reinfusion. In one or two of these cases there was a marked haemolysis, which could explain the finding, but in the other cases we could find no satisfactory explanation.

Does it matter if maximal aerobic power can be increased by a few per cent? Firstly, it should be borne in mind that in sport the difference in performance between first and last, in a top-level event, may be only measurable in parts of a per cent, which means that even very small changes in the different factors contributory to physical performance may be of vital importance. Secondly, increasing gross maximal aerobic power by 5 per cent in an already well-trained athlete may be almost impossible, at least over a year or so.

Figure 4.4 gives data for two well-trained athletes who were subjected to reinfusion of red blood cells. In one subject, resting heart rate on waking in the morning, and time on a 9 km cross-country test course are given. The arrow indicates the time of blood reinfusion. His best time before reinfusion was over a minute more than after the reinfusion. The other subject, a well-trained runner, reduced his best time by some 25–30 s on a hilly course. In both cases performance was increased dramatically and by about the same order of magnitude as in the laboratory experiments.

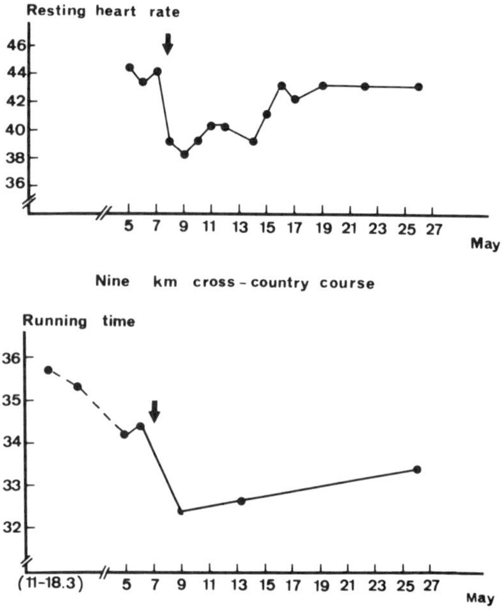

Fig. 4.4. Resting heart rate and running time following red blood cell reinfusion (marked with arrow) in two well-trained athletes.

In summary, it is with some regret that I conclude that our basic exercise physiology experiments on manipulation of haemoglobin concentration have some consequences for sport. It is undoubtedly clear – and confirmed by other groups (i.e. Buick *et al.* 1980) – that by increasing haemoglobin concentration maximal aerobic power will increase. Central circulation during maximal exercise is mainly unaffected by the reinfusion. The working muscle can evidently utilize the increased 'offered oxygen' and thus performance is increased.

References

Bergh, U., Kanstrup, I.-L., and Ekblom, B. (1976). Maximal oxygen uptake during exercise with various combinations of arm and leg work. *J. appl. Physiol.* **41**, 191–6.

Buick, F. J., Gledhill, N., Froese, A. B., Spriet, L., and Meyers, E. C. (1980). Effect of induced erythrocythemia on aerobic work capacity. *J. appl. Physiol: Respirat. Environ. Exercise Physiol.* **48**, 636–42.

Ekblom, B. and Hermansen, L. (1968). Cardiac output in athletes. *J. appl. Physiol.* **25**, 619–25.

—— Goldbarg, A. N., And Gullbring, B. (1972). Response to exercise after blood loss and reinfusion. *J. appl. Physiol.* **33**, 175–80.

—— Wilson, G., and Åstrand, P. O. (1976). Central circulation during exercise after venesection and reinfusion of red blood cells. *J. appl. Physiol.* **40**, 379–83.

Gullbring, B., Holmgren, A., Sjöstrand, T., and Strandell, T. (1960). The effects of blood volume variations on the pulse rate in supine and upright position and during exercise. *Acta physiol. scand.* **50**, 62–71.

Robinson, B. F., Epstein, S. E., Kahler, R. L., and Braunwald, E. (1966). Circulatory effects of acute expansion of blood volume. *Circulation Res.* **19**, 26–32.

Rowell, L. B. (1962). Factors affecting the prediction of maximal oxygen intake from measurements made during submaximal work with observations related to factors which may limit oxygen intake. Thesis. University of Minnesota, Minneapolis, MN.

Spriet, L. L., Gledhill, N., Froese, A. B., Wilkes, D. L ., and Meyers, E. C. (1980). The effect of induced erythrocythemia on central circulation and oxygen transport during maximal exercise. *Med. Sci. Sports Abstr.* **12**, 122.

Williams, M. H., Goodwin, A. R., Perkins, R., and Bocrie, J. (1973). Effect of blood reinjection upon endurance capacity and heart rate. *Med. Sci. Sports* **5**, 181–6.

5 Women in sport

M. O'BRIEN, B. DAVIES, AND A. DAGGETT

Introduction

With the increase in recreational opportunity, the active participation of women in sport has gathered momentum during the last decade. Inevitably, interest has developed in the physiological responses of females to these activites (Jordan 1977; Runyan and Puhl 1980; Mayhew, Piper, and Etheridge 1979) and the effects of these activities on the participants (Dale, Detlef, Gerlach, and Wilhite 1979a; Wentz 1980). Of particular concern has been the quantitative and qualitative differences between the sexes in their physiological responses to activities (Mayhew 1977; Cureton and Sparling 1980; Massicote, Avon, and Corriveau 1979).

Anthropometric considerations

To speak in terms of the 'woman athlete' is inappropriate. As the range of sporting activities has widened, it has become apparent that each event has participants with anthropometric and performance characteristics that uniquely describe the competitors (Carter 1981; Novak, Woodward, Bestit, and Mellerowicz 1977; Slaughter, Lohman, Riner, and Boileau 1980). Studies describing the anthropometric and performance characteristics of highly skilled athletes (Krahenbuhl, Wells, Brown, and Ward 1979; Malina, Harper, Avent, and Campbell 1971; Morrow, Hosler, and Nelson 1980; Spence, Disch, Fred, and Coleman 1980) have highlighted the importance of obtaining normative data for each event, in order to classify athletes.

It has been proposed that the anthropometric prototype for success exists in many sports based upon somatotype, body composition, and absolute and relative body dimensions (Hudson 1980). Although over the last half century the sociological trends which influence the status of male competitors have stabilized, this is not the case for women. The female athlete is relatively similar to her male counterpart in those anthropometric variables with a high genetic component, e.g. maximum oxygen uptake, and more dissimilar on those variables with a high environmental component, e.g. training regimens. It is expected, therefore, that training programmes might be devised that would eventually mould female athletes to a prototype which is modelled on the elite male performer.

The normal female has 46 chromosomes, 44 autosomal and XX; the male sex chromosomes are XY. There are a variety of chromosomal abnormalities, among them Klinefelter's syndrome XXY, Turner's syndrome XO, and XXX – the so called 'super female'. Individuals may also have a mosaic pattern, the cells containing chromosomes which have developed from two or more stem lines. All females competing in the Olympic Games and in International competitions must undergo a sex test. Problems arise if an individual has a chromosome abnormality, or the rarer testicular feminization syndrome (Lennox 1968) when the individual has XY sex chromosomes, has testes, but looks and acts as a female.

Strength

General muscle strength in the female has been estimated as being two thirds that of the male (Hettinger 1961). In terms of absolute strength, women are weaker in the upper body (Wilmore 1974; Montoye and Lamphiear 1977) but similar in lower body strength (Wilmore 1974; Hoffman, Stauffer, and Jackson 1979). Wilmore (1974) reports that leg strength is actually slightly greater in the female when related to units of lean body weight. Similarly, Ikai and Fukanaga (1968) have shown that the force exerted by equally sized muscles is the same in both sexes. As a consequence of such studies, it has been suggested that the well-trained female might be stronger than the untrained male (Harris 1977) and would, therefore, have a comparable or better strength/weight ratio. Morrow and Hosler (1981) do not support this contention. In utilizing isokinetic, as well as isometric and isotonic strength measures, they found significant differences between males and females in upper and lower body strengths. Although the distribution curves for absolute strength overlapped, showing that some women were, in fact, stronger than men, overall the males were stronger. Substantial gains in strength have been observed in both trained and untrained females, following weight training programmes (Brown and Wilmore 1974). Gains in muscle strength are accompanied by a less pronounced increase in the size of the muscle fibres than occurs in males. Muscle hypertrophy appears to be regulated in adult males and females by testosterone, which is found in much greater levels in males than in females (Wilmore 1975). Krahenbuhl, Archer, and Petit (1978) found no relationship between serum testosterone and strength in females, but the compensatory changes which accompany training and improve oxygen transport were greater in subjects with a high level of serum testosterone. This supports the theory that testosterone may play a significant role in the trainability of females. Dale, Detlef, Gerlach, Martin, and Alexander, (1979b) have demonstrated that serum testosterone levels are significantly higher in runners than in members of their control groups.

Muscle fibre composition expressed as the percentage of slow twitch fibres is slightly lower in women than in men (Karlsson 1980). Komi (1980) has found that isometric leg-extension strength of women is 80 per cent that of their male counterparts and, similarly, muscular power and maximal running velocity are 68 per cent and 85 per cent respectively, of the values for men. He suggests that the primary reason for the reduced muscular power in females can be attributed to their lower neuro-motor efficiency in combination with qualitatively and quantitatively different skeletal muscle.

The theory that females may be able to utilize a greater portion of their stored elastic energy in jumping activities gains support from Komi and Bosco (1978). During all experimental conditions, men were able to jump higher and sustain greater stretch loads than women. However, examination of the utilization of elastic energy indicated that, in jumps which allowed a counter movement, female subjects were able to utilize most (≙ 90 per cent) of the energy produced in the pre-stretching phase, in comparison to the 50 per cent of that of their male counterparts.

Anatomical differences

Women tend to be smaller and lighter than males and have a lower centre of gravity. The centre of gravity is usually in the region of sacral (S1) and in women is 55 per cent of standing height while in males it is 56–57 per cent (Blanksby 1973).

The female pelvis differs from that of the male in many particulars and the distinctive sex characteristics are already present in the foetal pelvis by the third or fourth month of intrauterine life (Boucher 1957). The female pelvis is wider in all its diameters, particularly the inferior aspect; the pelvic cavity is rounder, roomier, shorter, and less funnel-shaped than that of the male; the sacrum is shorter, wider, and less curved (James and Brubaker 1973). The sub-pubic angles are greater than 90° in the female. The acetabulum is smaller in the female but the distance between the acetabulum and the pubic symphysis is greater, thus increasing the width of the pelvis. Because of the wider pelvis in the female, there is a greater tendency to genu valgum or knocked knees; the normal pull of the quadriceps tends to pull the patella laterally, a tendency magnified by the wider pelvis, and chrondromalacia patella is relatively common. Research suggests that relationships between width of hips and running speed is low and should not be an inhibiting factor (Oyster and Wooten 1971; Thomas 1974). The shoulders are narrower and the bones of the upper limbs are shorter in the female. The carrying angle, measured when the forearm is fully extended, the hand is supinated, and the forearm is directed laterally is 167° in female and 173° in male. The angle disappears on flexion of the elbow, but it is a disadvantage to females in throwing events.

Body composition

The average female has twice as much measurable fat as the average male (De Vries 1981); 20–25 per cent for females compared to 10–14 per cent for males. There is also a wide variation amongst trained female athletes. Novak *et al.* (1977) found swimmers to have relatively more fat (18 per cent) than runners and gymnasts (13.3 and 12.9 per cent, respectively). Distribution of the subcutaneous fat showed that the swimmers had greater fat deposits over biceps, on the forearm, calf, iliac crest, and around the umbilicus, but not so the thighs or subscapular. However, gymnasts differed from runners, having more fat deposited on the biceps. It is well documented that the trained female has relatively less fat than normal sedentary controls (Novak *et al.* 1977; Dale *et al.* 1979a; Morrow *et al.* 1980). The lowest reported value for an athlete is six per cent (Brown and Wilmore 1974).

The idea that the percentage body fat is related to the onset and continued maintenance of menstrual cycle function has been proposed by Frisch (1977). Carlberg, Buckman, Peake, and Riedesel (1981) reported all runners covering distances greater than 55 miles per week, and weighing less than 100 per cent ideal body weight, to be amenorrhoeic. Dale *et al.* (1979a) suggest that there is probably no single amount of training weight-loss or per cent adipose tissue that will induce amenorrhoea in every woman, and points to the possibility of an individual amenorrhoeic threshold. However, the role of one critical value for body fat in menstrual rhythmicity remains uncertain. Recent studies (Hendrix and Lohman 1981; Snyder, Froehlich, and Lamb 1981) have not supported the hypothesis of a relationship between menstrual disorders and a critical body fat content, or maintenance of a particular ratio of fat to body weight in athletic populations. It appears more likely that weight loss is most closely correlated with the incidence of amenorrhoea (Knuth, Hull, and Jacobs 1977; Wentz 1980).

As body weight is lost, body fat is also lost; shifts in adipose tissue accompanying this may be critical. Loss of body weight in the range 10–15 per cent of normal weight and height, which represents a loss of one third of body fat, is said to result in amenorrhoea (Frisch, Revelle, and Cook 1973). Dale *et al.* (1979b) found that runners who were 13 pounds below average weight for height, had significantly less body fat, and had lost 5.9 per cent of their body weight since the onset of training. Athletes with the most intensive training schedules, and those who had been running for the longest time, had a higher incidence of oligo/amenorrhoea than their jogging and non-running controls.

Return of normal menses has been noted by Knuth *et al.* (1977) following simple weight gain, and by Erdelyi (1976) and Dale *et al.* (1979b) when training is reduced. Whether return of menses is caused by decreased training or increased deposition of adipose tissue remains uncertain. Of particular significance to sportswomen is the occasional decrease in body weight after discontinuing the use of oral contraceptives, and the corresponding increase in amenorrhoea (Dale *et al.* 1979b). The excretion of oestrogen varies with body weight and amount of fat; changes in body fat can alter the pathway of oestrogen metabolism (Fishman, Boyar, and Hellman 1975). Following oral contraception, where weight loss occurs with the decrease in body fat, there is occasionally an inability to resume normal oestrogen metabolic pathways.

Running performance

The greater average relative fat of females compared to males has been proposed as one of the factors responsible for the sex differences in distance running performances (Wilmore, Brown, and Davis 1977; Cureton, Hensley, and Tiburzi 1979). The latter utilized externally added weights to the trunks of a group of males which equated the extra percentage of body-fat weight of a group of matched females. The result was to reduce the mean sex differences in performance for a 12-minute run by 32 per cent. These investigations suggest that the primary metabolic consequence of the greater amount of body fat of the female is the increase in energy required to run at any given speed, therefore requiring a greater per cent of $V_{O_2\ max}$ and greater physiological stress. In elite male and female runners, who differ less in running economy, sex differences in percentage of fat may be of greater relative importance. In swimming, sex differences in body composition tend to be advantageous, the reduction in body drag leading to less energy expenditure per unit of distance swum (Pendergast, Wilson, di Prampero, and Rennie 1974). When maximum oxygen uptake measured on a bicycle ergometer is expressed in relation to fat-free weight or active muscle mass, sex differences have been observed to be virtually eliminated (Davies, Barnes, and Godfrey 1972).

It is interesting to speculate upon the other factors which might influence performance. For example, the average fibre diameter appears to be less than that in the male in both trained and untrained females, as is the capillary density per fibre ratio (Ingjer and Brodal 1978).

In the same study, although capillary density was found to be similar in both males and females, a maximum oxygen uptake ($\dot{V}_{O_2\ max}$) difference of 15 per cent was observed in favour of the males. Differences between untrained and endurance-trained females were evident in fibre diameter, number of capillaries per fibre, and capillary density, and were similar to the findings in males (Brodal, Ingjer, and Hermansen 1977). These differences must be, in part, due to training.

Although there is little doubt that the average $\dot{V}O_{2\,max}$ of the normal female is less than that of the normal male (Drinkwater 1973), the data suggest that the level of physical fitness of some groups of subects overrides the effect of sex differences. In particular, on the $\dot{V}O_{2\,max}$ scale, trained females overlap with untrained males. However, when comparing the mean $\dot{V}O_{2\,max}$ scores of trained athletes, differences of 20–28 per cent have been observed.

At similar submaximal loads, women are usually working at a higher percentage of their $\dot{V}O_{2\,max}$. Studies directly measuring sex differences in the aerobic demands of submaximal running have often been complicated by the difficulty of equating a group of male and female runners. Daniels, Krahenbuhl, Foster, Gilbert, and Daniels (1977) used highly-trained male and female runners to assess the aerobic elements of running at speeds ranging from 150 to 250 m/min, and observed no significant differences in the aerobic demands of running at submaximal speeds between males and females of relatively equal ability and fitness. Similarly, Mayhew *et al.* (1979) found the oxygen cost of running relative to body weight to be independent of sex and degree of training. The limit on the running speed of females appeared to be related to $\dot{V}O_{2\,max}$.

The differences in the circulatory adjustments to exercise do affect the ability of women to perform maximal or submaximal work. Smaller blood volumes and lower haemoglobin levels in women reduce the amount of oxygen available to the tissues; this must be compensated for at submaximal level by an increased cardiac output. At maximal level further compensation is limited by heart volume, blood volume, and venous return. When all responses are expressed in relation to a hypothetical work load of 50 per cent $\dot{V}O_{2\,max}$ (Åstrand and Rodahl 1970), cardiac output, stroke volume, and $\dot{V}O_{2\,max}$ are less, and heart rate is higher in women.

Although there have been many investigations of the structural and functional changes in the heart of male athletes, there is little information available on the female athlete. It is known that females have smaller hearts than males and this is reflected in their smaller left ventricular mass, left ventricular dimensions, and stroke volume. However, from studies involving a variety of athletic participants (Zeldis, Morganroth, and Rubler 1978; Rerych, Scholz, Sabiston, and Jones 1980), it would seem that women adapt to training in a similar manner to males. This is achieved by increases in left ventricular dimensions and wall thickness. More recent work (Rubal, Rosentsweig, and Hamerly, 1981), has shown significant differences between moderately endurance-conditioned games players and their controls, with changes in favour of the athletes in left ventricular diastolic dimension, diastolic volume, total left ventricular volume, left ventricular muscle volume, and muscle mass.

Anaerobic power

When anaerobic power is ascertained using a power test (Margaria, Aghemo, and Rovelli, 1966), there is very little difference between the sexes. Recent work involving short-term maximum exercise has highlighted some sex-related differences in the biochemical responses (Jacobs and Tesch 1980). It appears that differences exist in the interrelationships between short-term maximal exercise, muscle-fibre type distribution, lactate concentrations, and fatigue. In females, negative relationships were observed between percentage of fast-twitch muscle-fibre area and post-exercise muscle lactate, peak power, and post-exercise muscle lactate; and an insignificant relationship between lactate concentration and peak or average power. In contrast, males exhibited the reverse of the above. Karlsson (1980) has noted lower enzyme activity amongst females related to ATP splitting and regeneration from other energy-rich sources, such as creatine phosphate and glycogen.

Hagerman, Fox, Connors, and Pompei (1974) and Drinkwater, Horvath, and Wells (1975a) have documented lower levels of lactic acid following maximal exercise in females.

Iron metabolism

An area critical to the exercising female is iron metabolism. The lower oxygen-transport capacity of the female is known to affect female performance in endurance events. The oxygen-carrying capacity is similarly limited by the number of red blood cells (RBC) and the haemoglobin (Hb) concentration. Blood volume and Hb differences are approximately 25 per cent in untrained populations, and 12 per cent in trained athletes, in favour of the male. Post-menarchial females experience greater losses of body iron than the average male (Custer 1974) and trained women athletes have demonstrated lower serum iron levels (SeFe) than their sedentary counterparts (Haymes, Harris, Beldon, Loomis, and Nicholas 1972). A positive correlation between Hb and oxygen consumption has been demonstrated by Ekblom, Goldbarg, and Gullbring (1972) whereas, in terms of performance, Runyan and Puhl (1980) found no relationship with Hb and RBC's in their athletic population. Freedson, Katch, and Gilliam (1981) suggest that subjects with low Hb ($<$13.0 g/100 ml) counteract a reduced carrying capacity with greater quantities of 2, 3-diphosphoglycerate (2, 3-DPG) which enhances oxygen extraction. SeFe levels decrease only if iron cost exceeds storage. Iron costs appear to be associated with training (Bottiger, Nyberg, Åstrand, I. and Åstrand, P. O. 1971; Kilbom 1971), however, some subjects may have sufficient storage iron to absorb training effects (Writh, Lohman, Avallone, Shire, and Boileau 1978). Sub-normal levels of Hb indicate an advanced stage of serum iron deficiency. This has been demonstrated with athletes, who have exhibited a normal Hb during intensive training, with a corresponding low serum iron (Strauzenberg and Kabner 1980). These investigators advocate iron supplementation for female athletes. This has been endorsed by Ehn, Carlmark, and Hoglund (1980), who found significant improvement in Hb and ferritin levels in female athletes compared to their athletic controls. Nilson, Schoene, Robertson, Escourrov, and Smith (1981) gave iron therapy to minimally iron-deficient females. No improvement was observed on $\dot{V}O_{2\ max}$ or exercise time, but a reduction in maximum lactate level suggested that tissue iron plays a role in anaerobic metabolism. Tissue iron depletion, unrelated to anaemia, may therefore enhance lactate production and muscle fatigue during intensive exercise.

Training

The acute and chronic physiological effects of training have been well documented in men. Comparisons between the sexes have, in the main, been made from studies dealing exclusively with each sex, but a few authors (Massicote *et al.* 1979) have included both males and females in their studies. The evidence suggests that there are no differences between the sexes on adaptation to training (Kilbom 1971; Flint, Drinkwater, and Horvath 1974; Cunningham and Hill 1975). However, Lesmes, Fox, Stevens, and Otto (1978) found $\dot{V}O_2$ changes in females to be independent of intensity, following high-intensity interval training of different frequencies. Their study was in conflict with similar studies using men.

Detraining

Eriksson, Lunding, and Saltin (1975) have postulated that there are no beneficial effects from previous levels of training, preceding a number of years detraining. Pederson and Jorgensen (1978) have shown that detraining over a seven-week period is sufficient to neutralize the effect of a conditioning programme in women. Following supramaximal training (Weltman, Moffatt, and Stamford 1978), improvements in anaerobic power output, anaerobic capacity, and aerobic power were observed. However, detraining removed the aerobic improvement, with the anaerobic responses, particularly anaerobic power, remaining elevated. No such changes were observed in a control group. Drinkwater *et al.* (1975a) have shown the decrease in $\dot{V}O_{2\ max}$ after detraining to be less in trained athletes than their sedentary counterparts.

Thermoregulatory responses

It is generally accepted that sex differences exist in response to heat stress. Men commence sweating at lower skin temperatures and show higher sweat rates at equivalent body temperatures (Fox, Lofstedt, Woodward, and Eriksson 1969). Despite an apparent advantage in favour of men, women are able to regulate their body temperature with a lower sweat rate (Morimoto, Slabochova, Naman, and Sargent 1967). Since a significant number of the world's female athletic population participate under conditions of heat and humidity, it is not uncommon for women to exercise in a hypohydrated state. Byrd, Stewart, Torranin, and Berringer (1977) noted no sex differences following moderate levels of hypohydration in physiological responses to exercise. Some studies have highlighted a lesser degree of heat tolerance in women. It is thought, however, that much of the difference might be accounted for by the lower degree of physical fitness of the females (Wyndham, Morrison, and Williams 1965). When the work has been equated, the females' response is similar to that of the males. It would seem that sex, *per se*, is a small factor, when assessing the causes of thermal stress in relation to body size, physical fitness, and state of acclimatization (Nunnerley 1978). Trained women show greater stability and respond to moderate dehydration in the same way as men (Drinkwater, Denton, Kupprat, Talag, and Horvath 1975b; Drinkwater, Kupprat, and Horvath 1977), with the menstrual cycle having little effect on performance.

Recent work of Dill, Soholt, McLean, Drost, and Loughran (1977), has shown that the superior capacity of males for sustained exercise in desert heat was related to their higher aerobic capacity. Similarly, Drinkwater *et al.* (1975b) suggest that the superiority of trained over untrained women, when exercising at 48 °C, was related to their ability to maintain an adequate cardiac output. Anaerobically, no apparent sex differences between children have been observed during the Wingate test under three climatic conditions (Doton and Bar-Or 1980). However, Inbar, Doton, and Bar-Or (1980) have noted sex differences in the pattern of acclimatization to work in hot/dry conditions. It would seem that our current understanding of thermo-regulation is based on male populations; studies on women have been rare, and have usually involved only small numbers of subjects.

The menstrual cycle

There is marked disagreement amongst athletes on the effects of the menstrual cycle on performance (Zaharieva 1965). Variations in physical parameters at specific phases of the menstrual cycle have been studied over many years; yet confusion has arisen when interpreting the results of these studies, because the majority of investigators have not included gonadotropin and ovarian hormone analysis. In recent years, several studies have been completed (Shangold 1979; Davies and Daggett 1980; Bonen, Ling, MacIntyre, Neil, and McGrail 1979; Jurkowski, Jones, Walker, Younglai, and Sutton, 1978) which enable a more accurate study of the effects of the menstrual cycle on performance to be made, by verification of the occurrence of ovulation. Ovarian and gonadotropin hormones have well-defined characteristic patterns during the normal menstrual cycle (Speroff and Vandewiele 1971). Jurkowski *et al.* (1978) examined the effects of exercise intensity at specific phases of the cycle. Increases in progesterone (P), estradiol (E_2), and follicle-stimulating hormone (FSH) were noted; the latter in the follicular phase only, and P and E_2 increases during the luteal phase. Increases were dependent on the intensity of the exercise. Bonen *et al.* (1979) have observed similar results for E_2, with P rising at greater intensities and no change in FHS, prior to an exercise programme, with no changes in P and E_2, following the programme. An increased endurance time on the treadmill, at 90 per cent $\dot{V}O_{2\ max}$, has also been found during the luteal phase by Jurkowski *et al.* (1978). This may have implications for athletes in competition. The ovaries may be more sensitive to exercise during this phase of the cycle, thus increasing the release of the ovarian hormones. Performance might, therefore, be influenced by substrate metabolism (Bonen *et al.*1979), with lower exchange during the luteal phase. The greater oxidation of fatty acids retards the utilization of glycogen and lactate production (Costill, Coyle, Dalsky, Evans, Fink, and Hoopes 1977), possibly delaying the onset of fatigue.

No significant changes in performance during selected phases of the menstrual cycle have been found, following treadmill running at speeds ranging from 133 to 183 m/min (40–90 per cent of $\dot{V}O_{2\ max}$), in a group of active females (Davies and Daggett 1980).

The effects of chronic training on the ovarian and gonadotropin hormones have been studied (Bonen, Belcastro, Simpson, and Ling 1978) in young swimmers, who demonstrated depressed FSH levels and short luteal phases. Similarly, Bonen, Ling, Neil, and McGrail (1977) found consistently depressed FSH levels in normal subjects following training. Shangold *et al.* (1979) demonstrated decreased progesterone levels in the luteal phase over eighteen separate cycles during distance running (20–25 miles per week). It was noted that running during the luteal phase had a direct effect on that part of the cycle. The reduced progesterone levels were possibly due to decreased production, increased metabolism, or clearance. The data provide evidence for possible causes of infertility amongst distance runners, but the incidence amongst the athletic population as a whole has yet to be established.

It has been well recognized that oral contraceptive activates (OCA) will produce changes in haemostatic mechanisms (Hedlin, Milojevic, and Korey 1978). Similarly, the exercise effect on these mechanisms, namely, acceleration of clotting time (Poller, Priest, and Thomson 1971), increases in fibrinolytic activity (Cash 1966), and alterations in platelet number (Sarjas 1976) have been reported. It has been postulated (Hedlin *et al.* 1978) that the combination of OCA and exercise-induced changes may be different to those of exercise alone. It was found that although OCA did induce certain changes – raised fibrinogen and plasminogen levels, shorter recalcified clotting and dilute whole blood lysis time, and lower anti-thrombin – the OCA-induced changes did not diminish the exercise-induced changes. Seemingly, different pathways are available for these changes (Semar, Skoza, and Johnson 1969). The results suggest that oral contraceptive (OC) use probably does not reduce the possibility of benefit from exercise, because of the overriding effect of the latter. In demonstrating an increase in blood volume, stroke volume, and cardiac output during OC use, Lehtovirta, Kuikka, and Pyorala (1977) suggests that OCA could be an advantage to the female athlete. This argument gains support from the work of Ekblom *et al.* (1972) who demonstrated oxygen uptake and performance improvements as a result of hypervolaemia, brought about by auto-transfusion, and Rost, Hollmann, Liesen, and Schulten (1975) cited by Lehtovirta *et al.* (1977) who think that blood volume rather than Hb causes this change. In general, there is still confusion over the possible advantages or otherwise of OC use, largely because of the lack of long-term studies. One such study is that of Sandstrom, Backman, Dahlstrom, and Zador (1979) who noted increases in heart volume, blood pressure, and Hb during the first 12 months of OC use, with a reduced physical work capacity, only when related to Hb levels. After 12 months, all measurements returned to their pre-OCA levels, suggesting that an adaptive regulatory mechanism of the vascular system may play its part after a period of time.

Recent work (Haynes, Sopper, Wright, Low, Pierce, Graham, and Bonen 1981), has shown marked differences between controls and OC users in pre-exercise glucose levels and their exercise response at 40 and 80 per cent of maximum aerobic capacity. No differences were observed in free fatty acid, glycerol, or lactate levels.

It may be fair to conclude that the major difference in skeletal muscle and fat distribution will ensure that the superiority of males over females in general athletic performance will continue. However, it is also likely that more rigorous training regimes, in terms of intensity and commitment, for women athletes would reduce the present gap between male and female performance.

References

Åstrand, P. O. and Rodahl, K. (1970). *Textbook of work physiology*. McGraw-Hill, New York.

Blanksby, B. (1973). Biomechanics of swimming. *Int. Swimming (June)* 6–8.

Bonen, A., Ling, W., Neil, R., and McGrail, J. (1977). FSH, LH, progesterone and estradiol responses to exercise before and after training. *Can. J. appl. Sports Sci.* **2**, 225.
—— MacIntrye, K. P., Neil, R., McGrail, J. C., and Belcastro, A. N. (1979). Effect of exercise on serum concentrations of FSH, LH, progesterone and estradiol. *Eur. J. appl. Physiol.* **42**, 15–23.
—— Belcastro, A. N., Simpson, A. A., and Ling, W. Y. (1978). Comparisons of LH and FSH concentrations in age group swimmers on moderately active girls and adult women: The IVth Int. Conf. on Sports Sciences. *Swimming Med.* **6**, 70–8.
Bottiger, L. E., Nyberg, A., Åstrand, I., and Åstrand, P. O. (1971). Iron administration to healthy, physically very active students. *World Med.* **85**, 396–8.
Boucher, B. J. (1957). Sex differences in the foetal pelvis. *Am. J. Phys. Anthropol.* p. 58.
Brodal, P., Ingjer, F., and Hermansen, L. (1977). Capillary supply of skeletal muscle fibers in untrained and endurance-trained men. *Am. J. Physiol.* **232**, 705–12.
Brown, C. and Wilmore, J. (1974). The effects of maximal resistance training on the strength and body composition of women athletes. *Med. Sci. Sports* **6**, 174–77.
Byrd, R., Stewart, L., Torranin, C., and Berringer, O. M. (1977). Sex differences in response to hypohydration. *J. Sports Med.* **17**, 65–68.
Carlberg, K. A., Buckman, M. T., Peake, G. T., and Riedesel, M. L. (1981). Low body weight increases susceptibility to athletic oligo/amenorrhoea. *Med. Sci. Sports Exercise (ACSM 1981, Abstr.)* **13**, 105.
Carter, J. E. L. (1981). Size and somatotype of Olympic female athletes at Montreal. *Med. Sci. Sports Exercise (ACSM Annu. Meet.)* **13**, 2.
Cash, J. D. (1966). Effects of moderate exercise of fibrinolytic system in normal young men and women. *Br. Med. J.* **11**, 502–6.
Costill, D. L ., Coyle, E., Dalsky, G., Evans, W., Fink, W., and Hoopes, D. (1977). Effects of elevated plasma FFA and insulin on muscle glycogen usage during exercise. *J. appl. Physiol.* **43**, 695–9.
Cunningham, D. A. and Hill, J. S. (1975). Effect of training and cardiovascular response to exercise in women. *J. appl. Physiol.* **39**, 891–5.
Cureton, K. J. and Sparling, P. B. (1980). Distance running performance and metabolic responses to running in men and women with excess weight experimentally equated. *Med. Sci. Sports Exercise* **12**, 288–94.
—— Hensley, L. D., and Tiburzi, A. (1979). Body fatness and performance differences between men and women. *Res. Q.* **50**, 333–40.
Custer, R. P. (1974). *An atlas of the blood and bone marrow*, pp. 30–50. Saunders, Philadelphia.
Dale, E., Detlef, H., Gerlach, D. F., and Wilhite, M. A. (1979a). Menstrual dysfunction in distance runners. *Int. J. Obstet. Gynecol.* **54**, 47–53.
—— Martin, D. E., and Alexander, R. W. (1979b). Physical fitness profiles and reproductive physiology of the female distance runner. *Phys. Sports Med.* (Jan.) 83–95.
Daniels, J., Krahebuhl, G., Foster, C., Gilbert, J., and Daniels, S. (1977). Aerobic responses of female distance runners to sub-maximal and maximal exercise. *Ann. N.Y. Acad. Sci.* **301**, 726–33.
Davies, C., Barnes, C., and Godfrey, S. (1972). Body composition and maximal exercise performance in children. *Hum. Biol.* **44**, 195–214.
Davies, B. and Daggett, A. (1980). Physiological responses to exercise during selected phases of the menstrual cycle. *Int. Cong. Women and Sport (Abstr.)*. Rome, p. 52.

De Vries, H. (1981). *Physiology of exercise for physical education and athletics*. 3rd edn. Saunders College Publishing.
Dill, D. B., Soholt, L. F., McLean, D. C., Drost, T. F., and Loughran, M. T. (1977). Capacity of young males and females for running in desert heat. *Med. Sci. Sports* **9**, 137–42.
Doton, R. and Baro-Or, O. (1980). Climatic heat stress and performance in the Wingate anaerobic test. *Eur. J. appl. Physiol.* **44**, 237–43.
Drinkwater, B. (1973). Physiological responses of women to exercise. In *Exercise and sport sciences reviews (ed. J. Wilmore)* Vol. 1, pp. 126–30. Academic Press, New York.
—— Horvath, S. and Wells, C. (1975a). Aerobic power of females aged 10–68. *J. Gerontol.* **30**, 385–94.
—— Denton, J. E., Kupprat, I. C., Talag, T. S., and Hovarth, S. M. (1975b). Aerobic power as a factor in women's response to work in hot environments. *J. Gerontol.* **30**, 385–94.
—— Kupprat, I. C., and Hovarth, S. M. (1977). Heat tolerance of female distance runners. *Ann. N.Y. Acad. Sci.* **301**, 777–92.
Ehn, E., Carlmark, B., and Hoglund, S. (1980). Effects of iron supplementation with haemoglobin iron on haemoglobin levels and ferritin in female athletes. *Int. Congr. Women and Sport* (Abstr.). Rome, p. 60.
Ekblom, B., Goldbarg, A. N., and Gullbring, B. (1972). Response to exercise after blood loss and re-infusion. *J. appl. Physiol.* **33**, 175–80.
Erdelyi, G. J. (1976). Effects of exercise on the menstrual cycle. *Phys. Sports Med.* **4**, 79.
Eriksson, B., Lunding, A., and Saltin, B. (1975). Cardiopulmonary function in former girl swimmers and the effect of training on circulatory response to exercise. *Scand. J. clin. Lab. Invest.* **35**, 135–45.
Fishman, J., Boyar, R. M., and Hellman, L. (1975). Influence of body weight on estradiol metabolism in young women. *J. clin Endocr. Metab.* **41**, 989.
Flint, M. M., Drinkwater, B. L., and Hovarth, S. M. (1974). Effects of training on women's response to sub-maximal exercise. *Med. Sci. Sports* **6**, 89–94.
Fox, R. H., Lofstedt, B. E., Woodward, P. M., and Eriksson, E. (1969) Comparison of thermoregulatory function in men and women. *J. appl. Physiol.* **26**, 444–453.
Freedson, P. S., Katch, V. L., and Gilliam, T. B. (1981). The influence of haemoglobin concentration on sub-maximum exercise cardiac output: evidence of exercise intensity threshold. *Med. Sports Exercise (ACSM 1981 Conf., Abstr.)* **13**, 109.
Frisch, R. E. (1977). Fatness and the onset and maintenance of menstrual cycle. *Res. Reprod.* **6**, 1.
—— Revelle, R., and Cook, S. (1973). Components of the critical weight at menarche and at initiation of the adolescent sport: estimated total water, lean body mass and fat. *Hum. Biol.* **45**, 469.
Hagerman, F., Fox, E., Connors, M., and Pompei, J. (1974). Metabolic responses of women rowers during ergometric rowing. *Med. Sci. Sports* **6**, 87.
Harris, D. V. (1977) The female athlete: strength endurance and performance. In *Towards an Understanding of Human Performance* (ed. E. J. Burke), pp. 41–44. Ithaca and NY Movement, New York.
Haymes, E. M., Harris, D. V., Beldon, M. D., Loomis, J. L., and Nicholas, W. C. (1972). The effect of the physical activity level on selected hematological variables in adult women. *AAHPER* Abstr. 16.

Haynes, F., Sopper, M., Wright, W. W., Low, M., Pierce, G., Graham, T., and Bonen, A. (1981). Substrate and hormonal responses during exercise in users and non-users of oral contraceptives. *Med. Sci. Sports Exercise (ACSM Annu. Meet. Abstr.)* **13**, 105.

Hedlin, A. M., Milojevic, S., and Korey, A. (1978). Hemostatic changes induced by exercise during oral contraceptive use. *Can. J. Physiol. Pharmacol.* **56**, 316–20.

Hendrix, M. K. and Lohman, T. G. (1981). Incidence of menstrual disorders in female collegiate athletes and its relation to body fat content. *Med. Sci. Sports Exercise (ACSM 1981 Conf. Abstr.)* **13**, 104.

Hettinger, T. (1961). *Physiology of strength.* Thomas, Springfield, Ill.

Hoffman, T., Stauffer, R. W., and Jackson, A. S. (1979). Sex differences in strength. *Am. J. Sports Med.* **7**, 265–267.

Hudson, J. (1980). The anthropometric prototype of the elite female athlete. *Inst. Cong. Women and Sport (Abstr.)* , Rome, p. 89.

Ikai, M. and Fukanaga, T. (1968). Calculations of muscle strength per unit cross-sectional area of human muscle by means of ultrasonic measurements. *Int. Z. Angew. Physiol.* **26**, 26–32.

Inbar, O., Doton, R., and Bar-Or, O. (1980). Acclimatization to dry heat: a comparison between men and women. *Int. Cong. Women and Sport.* (Abstr.), Rome, p. 90.

Ingjer, F. and Brodal, P. (1978). Capillary supply of skeletal muscle fibres in untrained and endurance trained women. *Eur. J. appl. Physiol.* **38**, 291–299.

Jacobs, I. and Tesch, P. (1980). Short time, maximal muscular performance – relation to muscle lactate and fibre type in females. *Int. Congr. on Women and Sport (Abstr.).* Rome, p. 194.

James, S. and Brubaker, C. (1973). Biochemical and neuromuscular aspects of runners. In *Exercise and sports science reviews* (ed. J. Wilmore), Vol. 1, pp. 189–216. Academic Press, New York.

Jordan, D. B. (1977). Analysis of exercise stress test and responses of adult marathon runners. *J. Sport Med. Phys. Fitness* **17**, 59–64.

Jurkowski, J. E., Jones, L. N., Walker, W. C., Younglai, E. V., and Sutton, J. R. (1978). Ovarian hormonal responses to exercise. *J. appl. Physiol.* **44**, 109–14.

Karlsson, J. (1980). Skeletal muscle fibre characteristics in males and females. *Int. Congr. Women and Sport (Abstr.)*, Rome, p. 100.

Kilbom, A. (1971). Physical training in women. *Scand. J. clin. Lab. Invest.* **28**, 141–61.

Knuth, V. A., Hull, M. G. R., and Jacobs, H. S. (1977). Amenorrhoea and loss of weight. *Br. J. Obstet. Gynaecol.* **84**, 80L.

Komi, P. V. (1980). Fundamental performance characteristics in females and males. *Int. Congr. Women and Sport (Abstr.)*, Rome, p. 103.

—— and Bosco, C. (1978). Utilization of stored elastic energy in leg extensor muscles by men and women. *Med. Sci. Sports* **10**, 261–5.

Krahenbuhl, G. S., Archer, L., and Petit, L. L. (1978). Serum testosterone and adult female trainability. *J. Sports Med.* **18**, 359–64.

—— Wells, C. L., Brown, C. H., and Ward, P. E. (1979). Characteristics of national and world class female pentathletes. *Med. Sci. Sports* **11**, 20–3.

Lehtovirta, P., Kuikka, J., and Pyorala, T. (1977). Hemodynamic effects of oral contraceptives during exercise. *Int. J. Gynacol. Obstet.* **15**, 35–7.

Lennox, B. (1968). Some observations on the difficulty of determining sex. *Bull. Br. Assoc. Sports Med.* **3**, 80.

Lesmes, G. R., Fox, E. L., Stevens, C., and Otto, R. (1978). Metabolic responses of females to high intensity interval training of different frequencies. *Med. Sci. Sports* **10**, 229–32.

Malina, R. M., Harper, A. B., Avent, H. H., and Campbell, D. E. (1971). Physique of female track and field athletes. *Med. Sci. Sports* **3**, 32–8.

Margaria, R., Aghemo, P., and Rovelli, E. (1966). Measurement of muscular power (anaerobic) in man. *J. appl. Physiol.* **21**, 1664.

Massicotte, D. R., Avon, G., and Corriveau, G. (1979). Comparative effects of aerobic training on men and women. *J. Sports Med.* **19**, 23–32.

Mayhew, J. L. (1977). Oxygen cost and energy expenditure of running in trained runners. *Br. J. Sports Med.* **11**, 116–21.

—— Piper, F. C., and Etheridge, M. A. (1979). Oxygen cost and energy requirement of running in trained and untrained males and females. *J. Sports Med.* **19**, 39–44.

Montoye, H. J. and Lamphiear, D. E. (1977). Grip and arm strength in males and females aged 10–69. *Res. Q.* **48**, 109–120.

Morimoto, T., Slabochova, Z., Naman, R. K., and Sargent, F. (1967). Sex differences in physiological reaction to thermal stress. *J. appl. Physiol.* **22**, 526–32.

Morrow, J. R. and Hosler, W. W. (1981). Strength comparison in untrained men and trained women athletes. *Med. Sci. Sports Exercise* **13**, 194–8.

—— —— and Nelson, J. K. (1980). A comparison of women intercollegiate basketball players, volleyball players and non-athletes. *J. Sports Med.* **20**, 435–40.

Nilson, K., Schoene, R. B., Robertson, H. T., Escourrov, P., and Smith, N. J. (1981). The effect of iron repletion on exercise-induced lactate production in minimally iron-deficient subjects. *Med. Sci. Sports Exercise (ACSM Annu. Meet. Abstr.)* **13**, 92.

Novak, L. P., Woodward, W. A., Bestit, C., and Mellerowicz, H. (1977). Working capacity, body composition and anthropometry of olympic female athletes. *J. Sports Med.* **17**, 275–83.

Nunnerley, S. A. (1978). Physiological responses of women to thermal stress: a review. *Med. Sci. Sports* **10**, 250–5.

Oyster, N. and Wooten, E. (1971). The influence of selected anthropometric measurements on the ability of college women to perform the 35 yard dash. *Med. Sci. Sports* **3**, 130–4.

Pederson, P. K. and Jorgensen, K. (1978). Maximal oxygen uptake in young women with training, inactivity and retraining. *Med. Sci. Sports* **10**, 233–7.

Pendergast, D., Wilson, D., di Prampero, P., and Rennie, D. (1974). Energy cost of swimming. *Med. Sci. Sports* **6**, 86.

Poller, L., Priest, C. M., and Thomson, J. M. (1971). Platelet aggregation and strenuous exercise. *J. Physiol., Lond.* **213**, 525–31.

Rerych, S. K., Scholz, D. M., Sabiston, D. C., and Jones, R. H. (1980). Effects of exercise training on left ventricular function in normal subjects: a longitudinal study by radionuclide angiography. *Am. J. Cardiol.* **45**, 244–52.

Rost, R., Hollmann, W., Liesen, H., and Schulten, D. (1975). Cited by Lehtovirta, P., Kuikka, J., and Pyorala, T. (1977). Hemodynamic effects of oral contraceptives during exercise. *Int. J. Gynaecol. Obstet.* **15**, 35–7.

Rubal, B. J., Rosentsweig, J., and Hamerley, B. (1981). Echocardiographic examination of women collegiate softball champions. *Med. Sci. Sports Exercise* **13**, 176–9.

Runyan, W. S. and Puhl, J. (1980). Relationships between selected blood indices and competitive performance in college women cross-country runners. *J. Sports Med.* **20**, 207–12.

Sandstrom, B., Backman, C., Dahlstrom, J. A., and Zador, G. (1979). Adjustments of circulation including blood pressure to orthostatic reaction and physical exercise during application of a low oestrogen dose steroid oral contraceptive. *Acta. Obstet. Gynecol. Scand. Suppl.* **88**, 49–55.

Sarjas, H. S. S. (1976). Reaction patterns of blood platelets in exercise. *Adv. Cardiol.* **18**, 176–95.

Semar, M., Skoza, L., and Johnson, A. J. (1969). Partial purification and properties of plasminogen activator from human erythrocytes. *J. clin. Invest.* **48**, 1777–85.

Shangold, M. (1979). The relationship between long distance running and plasma progesterone, and luteal phase length. *Fertil. Steril.* **31**, 130–3.

Slaughter, M. H., Lohman, T. G., Riner, W. F., and Boileau, R. A. (1980). Differences in body physique among five groups of college women athletes. *Int. Congr. Women and Sport (Abstrs)*, Rome, p. 153.

Snyder, A. C., Froehlich, M. P., and Lamb, D. R. (1981). Body fat and menstrual history of college athletes. *Med. Sci. Sports Exercise (ACSM 1981 Conf., Abstr)* **13**, 104–5.

Spence, D. W., Disch, J. G., Fred, H. L., and Coleman, A. E. (1980). Descriptive profiles of highly skilled women volleyball players. *Med. Sci. Sports Exercise* **12**, 299–302.

Speroff, L. and Vandeweile, R. L. (1971). Regulation of the human menstrual cycle. *Am. J. Obstet.* **109**, 234–47.

Strauzenberg, S. E. and Kabner, R. (1980). Iron deficiency in female athletes. *Int. Cong. Women and Sport* (Abstracts). Rome, p. 160.

Thomas, C. (1974). Special problems of female athletes. In *Sport and medicine* (eds.) A. Ryan and F. Allman, pp. 347–73. Academic Press, New York.

Weltman, A., Moffatt, R. J., and Stamford, B. A. (1978). Supramaximal training in females: effects on aerobic power output, anaerobic capacity and aerobic power. *J. Sports Med.* **18**, 237–44.

Wentz, A. C. (1980). Body weight and amenorrhoea. *Int. J. Obstet. Gynecol.* **56**, 482–7.

Wilmore, J. (1974). Alterations in strength, body composition and anthropometric measurements consequent to a 10-week weight training program. *Med. Sci. Sport* **6**, 138.

—— (1975). Body composition and strength development. *J. Phys. Educ. Rec.* **46**, 38–40.

—— Brown, C. H., and Davis, J. A. (1977). Body physique and composition of the female distance runner. *Ann. N.Y. Acad. Sci.* **301**, 775.

Writh, J. C., Lohman, T. G., Avallone, J. P ., Shire, T., and Boileau, R. A. (1978). The effect of physical training on the serum iron levels of college-age women. *Med. Sci. Sports* **10**, 223–6.

Wyndham, C. H., Morrison, J. F., and Williams, C. G. (1965). Heat reactions of male and female caucasions. *J. appl. Physiol.* **20**, 357–64.

Zaharieva, E. (1965). Survey of sportswomen at Tokyo Olympics. *J. Sports Med. Phys. Fitness* **5**, 215–19.

Zeldis, S. M., Morganroth, J., and Rubler, S. (1978). Cardiac hypertrophy in response to dynamic conditioning in female athletes. *J. appl. Physiol.* **44**, 849–52.

6 The contribution of sports biomechanics

A. J. SMITH

What is sports biomechanics?

Biomechanics may be described as the mechanical engineering approach to the study of human movement. Such a bald statement is open to misunderstanding and the main purpose of this chapter is to explain it. In using this description, we imply that biomechanics has used, and will continue to find most valuable, the extensive body of theoretical and experimental techniques which are available to the professional mechanical engineer engaged in research and design.

On the theoretical side there are well-established, mathematical methods dealing with the motion and deformation of complex bodies and structures, the flow patterns and resistances associated with fluid motion, and the energy exchanges within and between systems. Whilst it has long been possible to set up mathematical equations describing such phenomena, the last 20 years have seen considerable progress in the numerical solution of the more difficult cases by the use of computers to handle repetitive calculations and large amounts of data. The behaviour of complex systems is thereby more fully understood and the restrictive simplifying assumptions, which once characterized engineering theory, are being removed.

The experimental techniques of mechanical engineering – direct measurement of the deformation and spatial motion of bodies, and of the forces acting on them – have always been of interest to engineers, and the last two decades have witnessed rapid advances in the necessary electronic instrumentation. Techniques for the measurement of small deformations in loaded materials, of velocity and acceleration, and of compressive, tensile, and shearing forces, have improved in precision and reliability.

Many of these engineering methods are relevant to the study of human movement and this chapter offers some examples of their application to the study of sporting performance.

To define the field in question more closely, sports biomechanics, viewed as the mechanical engineering approach to the sportsman's activity and his equipment, is concerned not only with the functioning of the human body in skilled performance, but with the response of the sports equipment to the performer's demands, and the interactions which take place between man and equipment. We are faced here with intriguing, but often difficult problems in the motion and deformation of bodies, both human and inanimate.

It is important that biomechanical experiments should interfere as little as possible with the free performance of the athlete, so the measuring instruments are required to be unobtrusive, yet capable of high accuracy. Fortunately, recent developments in instrumentation and data recording, to which engineers owe a considerable debt, are providing elegant methods for the measurement of rapidly fluctuating motion variables through small, reliable transducers.

Theoretical study of the force–motion relationships in sports biomechanics goes alongside the experimental techniques. At first sight, it may appear that an engineering representation of the movement patterns and internal processes of the human body, together with the interplay of forces between man and his equipment, can provide only a crude, unrealistic view of the subtleties of sporting activity. On reflection, however, it becomes apparent that the engineer has developed the ability to recognize the essential mechanics of a system and to write mathematical descriptions of its behaviour. He learns to make judicious simplifications, conceiving, first mentally and diagrammatically, and later, mathematically, a 'model' of the major factors determining the system's behaviour. The early stages of such 'modelling' are something of an art, though the validity of the assumptions incorporated into the model is usually checked by experiment. In such a way the main areas of engineering design theory have been established and biomechanics has, to its advantage, adopted a similar philosophy. Those who regard the mechanics of human movement as an offensively simplistic view of the wonders of human performance, should perhaps make a more serious study of the more advanced methods now being employed, and ponder the possible improvements to come.

None the less, the complexity of human motion does present many problems to the worker in sports biomechanics, and it is not surprising that much of the earlier research was concentrated on simpler activities such as level walking and running, where the influence of equipment and environment appear to be minimal. Such activities are important too, because they are fundamental to human existence. They have proved to be much more interesting and subtle than would at first be imagined, and many questions on the mechanics of human locomotion remain unanswered.

More elaborate, often three-dimensional, patterns of motion occur in gymnastics, trampolining, and diving, though again the effects of equipment and surroundings are often negligible, interest being centred on the performer alone when he is airborne. Interaction with the equipment does, however, occur in most sports, and Newton's Third Law reminds us that, as the performer applies forces to his equipment, it applies equal and opposite forces to the performer. This law expresses the essential type of interaction which sports biomechanics tries to investigate. Obvious examples occur in pole-vaulting, rowing, and skiing, but more detailed consideration of even

Table 6.1. Main areas of sports biomechanics activity

1.	Whole-body segmental models
2.	Kinematics of movement
3.	Force measurement
4.	Kinetic or force-motion analysis
5.	Motion of the centre of gravity
6.	Part-body models
7.	Equipment design
8.	Man–equipment interaction
9.	Feedback control
10.	Descriptive mechanics, or kinesiology
11.	Statistical studies
12.	Physiological studies

the track runner suggests that he responds to the frictional and flexural properties of his shoes and the track itself.

The scope of sports biomechanics

The list of topics in Table 6.1 covers the main areas of work in sports biomechanics, in terms of the theoretical and experimental methods currently employed in the field. In the next section, each topic is expanded upon, some research techniques are mentioned, and examples of relevant literature are quoted. A further section looks at skiing as a specific sport upon which much recreational, commercial, research, and teaching interest is centred. Referring first to Table 6.1, a dozen distinct, but by no means dissociated areas, may be recognized.

Discussion of the main areas

Whole-body segmental models

A starting-point in the mathematical representation, or 'modelling', of the whole human body in motion is the concept of segmental representation of the body masses. Changes in relative positions of the trunk, limbs, and head during a human motion imply that the spatial distribution of the masses forming the body is continuously changing. The body may be thought of as a system of interconnected masses; the connections are the main skeletal joints and the masses simulate the segments, lower leg, upper leg, forearm, and so on. If reasonably accurate values can be assigned to the masses and dimensions of the segments, then changes in mass-distribution, due to variations in body configuration, can be calculated, and the mass-centre (for all practical purposes the centre of gravity) can be estimated in position.

Determination of the masses and other mechanical properties of body segments began with some pioneer dissection of the frozen corpses of suicides around 100 years ago. The workers, Braune and Fischer (1889), did not seem to attract many research students and the work was virtually, and no doubt practically, interred, until the advent of the United States Astronautics Program. A need then arose for data on the activities of man in low- and zero-gravity conditions. The names of Dempster (1955), Whitsett (1963), and Hanavan (1964) appear on more modern researches into segmental models. Their work has provided sets of standard 'mean-man' segmental masses, mass-centre locations, and moments of inertia, for use in human dynamic studies.

In setting out on a biomechanical analysis, one is often torn between the more straightforward course of adopting the well-tried 'mean-man' data from astronautics and the more difficult option of making direct measurement of segmental mass on one's own subjects. As far as we know, nobody has yet frozen and sawn up a twentieth-century sportsman, but other less intrusive methods, such as immersion of the body segments in water and measurement of the displaced fluid, have been put forward. Combined with approximate figures on body density, these measurements provide estimates of the masses for a specific subject.

In some instances, suitable data on inertial properties may be obtained without recourse to the conceptual or actual division into segments. For example, the performer himself may be required to lie on a rigid board in a particular bodily configuration. Measurement of the supporting forces at the corners of the board enables the experimenter to compute the location of the body's centre of gravity for that position. Forms of pendulum test have also been proposed (e.g. Santschi, Dubois, and Omoto 1963) in which the body is strapped in the desired configuration, within a light frame, and the whole is allowed to oscillate about a horizontal axis (swinging pendulum) or a vertical axis (torsional pendulum). Such experiments can provide both the location of the centre of gravity and the moment of inertia for the whole human body. It seems, however, that such methods cannot be accurately employed to provide data on the individual segments.

The type of segmental model described above is no more than a technique for handling the varying mass distribution of the body. It does not attempt to deal with the action of muscles across joints, or the elasticity of human tissue. A much more comprehensive representation, of both body masses and internal actions, has been published by Hatze (1977).

Kinematics of movement

In mechanics, the study of motion in terms of spatial displacement and time, without reference to the forces causing the motion, is known as kinematics. In biomechanics, records of the body's configurational changes during a movement, together with the velocities and accelerations of the whole body or its segments, can provide insight into important features of a skilled action. The time history of a movement is often most conveniently recorded by the cine or television camera. Slow motion 'action replays' are popular because they reveal points which the unaided human eye cannot discern. Frame-by-frame analysis of a high-speed cine film of human activity is an extension of this process, and gives a vast quantity of information. Patterns of angular movement of the limbs, times and points of contact with the surroundings, and the co-ordination of actions of the various segments, may be studied. Fascinating detail is often revealed.

In biomechanics, however, purely visual assessment of kinematic data is but the first stage of knowledge. Structure of a more important kind may be discerned in measurements from the filmed records which are condensed in graphical form. Thus, displacement–time graphs for both linear and angular motions of the body segments, plots of knee-joint angle against hip-joint angle, and curves of velocity and acceleration against time during a movement, lead to deeper understanding of the logic underlying the motion.

For example, knee–hip and knee–ankle diagrams, relating angular measures of displacement at pairs of joints during a walk or run, have been proposed by Grieve (1968) and applied to several aspects of locomotion study with useful results.

Velocities and accelerations of the body in locomotion have also been estimated from cine-film study of running action (Margaria, Cerretelli, Aghemo, and Sassi 1963). At times, however, the detailed records obtained from film analysis are not appropriate. Interesting work has been carried out by direct measurement of speed, using a device similar to the 'radar speed-trap' to measure velocity changes of the whole body during sprinting (Vaughan and Matravers 1977). Acceleration may also be measured directly by accelerometers mounted on the body, but a thorough experimenter might check such direct measurement of velocity or acceleration against computations based on a film of the action.

It will be clear that cine film or video tape holds much more potential information on the details of body motion than can be given by specific measuring devices mounted on the body. A permanent record of a sporting performance is produced on film and the camera can, of course, be used without any impediment to the athlete. It is, therefore, the only recording technique permissible during most competitive events.

It must be noted that the computational procedures which provide velocity and acceleration values from displacement–time data are inherently liable to generate large errors. From a mathematical standpoint, these procedures for calculation of the rate-of-change of a variable, or numerical differentiation, are not to be recommended for accuracy. In biomechanics, however, the filming of skilled movement remains a most valuable working technique and as much information as possible should be squeezed from the film. To this end, thought has been given to the refinement of numerical differentiation techniques. Winter, Sidwall, and Hobson (1974), for instance, discuss the filtering of 'noise', or random error, from locomotion data, and Lees (1980) examines ways in which computational procedures may be selected, based on frequency analysis of displacement–time data. With the wider use of computer facilities, such methods, which often require extensive numerical calculation, may be handled with ease and the accuracy of velocity and acceleration values can be much improved.

Force measurement

The direct measurement of forces is of primary interest in biomechanics, because it is through the muscular production of force that the body is propelled and is able to act upon bodies outside itself. Forces which remain constant over an appreciable time may often be measured by simple lever-balance or spring-balance methods, but forces which vary rapidly call for more refined instruments. In these cases, biomechanics has employed strain gauges, force transducers, and force platforms, together with sensitive electronic recording gear.

Strain gauges measure minute deformations in a material under stress and it is often a short step to calculate from strain data the forces responsible for these deformations. Strain gauges designed primarily to measure bending deformations have been used to investigate the loadings on canoe paddles and horizontal gymnastic bars (J. Emmett, personal communication 1980; I. W. Graham, personal communication 1979).

Force transducers or load cells operate on a number of different principles, one useful form being based on the response of a piezo-electric crystal to variations in compressive force. All such devices can be calibrated to provide direct reading of force. The compact transducers now available may be fitted into the soles of boots, incorporated in weight-training equipment and, indeed, be applied reasonably easily at any point where two bodies make surface contact. Combined with miniature telemetric transmitters, force transducers can transmit information on rapidly varying forces in high speed motion, such as those occurring between boot and binding in fast downhill skiing (Hull and Mote 1978).

The force platform is, in effect, an extremely rigid and sensitive weighing machine. Its most useful form is a rectangular plate let into a smooth floor, with no appreciable gaps or steps at the edges, so that the performer may walk, run, or jump on or off the platform. As he makes contact, sensitive pick-ups, usually strain gauges or other force transducers, mounted beneath and effectively supporting the platform, measure the variations in thrust. Many force platforms have been laboratory built, but there are commercial models, such as that manufactured by Kistler Instruments Limited.

The force platform is particularly valuable for the study of human locomotion, the vertical foot thrust being accurately recorded as the performer walks or runs over the platform. Many platforms measure forward and transverse components of horizontal force at the foot, as well as the vertical thrust. Studies of jumping have also been undertaken. The pattern of foot thrust is directly related to the success of the jumper in raising his centre of gravity, and may help to distinguish between good and poor styles of jumping.

The Force Platform Users' Association, centred on the Department of Physical Education at Birmingham University, collates information on platform design and applications.

Kinetic or force–motion analysis

Kinetics is the study of motion of bodies which relates the motion to the forces causing it. An important body of theory in mechanics is built on Newton's Second Law:

Force equals mass times acceleration

or in the more general form:

Force equals rate-of-change of momentum.

In biomechanics a combination of data from a segmental model and from the kinematics of motion allows computation of 'mass times acceleration' quantities for the body segments. With these 'inertia forces', and an application of Newton's Second Law, external forces associated with a motion pattern may be deduced.

As an example, consider the standing vertical jump. The modest jumper can raise his centre of gravity some 15 inches, whilst the good performer produces a lift of over 30 inches. Side-view cine filming provides information on the segmental motions, which are essentially in the vertical plane (a judicious assumption, which might later be checked). Frame-by-frame measurement of segment positions provides displacement–time histories, from which velocities and accelerations of the segments may be calculated. Summation of the 'mass times vertical acceleration' products for all segments gives a total inertia force and it is a simple matter to apply Newton's Second Law to obtain the varying vertical foot thrust during the period before take-off. This force pattern is directly related to the velocity of take-off and, hence, the height achieved by the jumper.

Alongside this method for computing the force–time history, a second totally independent record may be obtained by having the performer jump from a force platform. A calculated thrust variation may be suspect, despite refined error-smoothing procedures and it is, therefore, desirable to compare the computed force with one measured directly. If reasonable agreement is obtained, then the film analysis procedures are largely validated (e.g. Smith 1972). An important consequence of such validation is that reliable estimation may be made of forces within the body which cannot be measured by direct methods. Values of force at the knee-joint, for instance, may be estimated by using Newton's Second Law on a part, rather than the whole, of the body, an imaginary section being made at the knee.

Extensive use of film analysis and computer methods for the evaluation of forces and moments at the major joints during a wide range of sports activities will be found in Plagenhoef (1971).

Motion of the centre of gravity

Some important features of a motion are made clear when the movement of the centre of gravity of the body is determined. Newton's Second Law in the form:

Sum of external forces equals mass times acceleration of the centre of gravity

may be applied to any body, and is particularly valuable when the body in question is continually changing shape during the motion. The springboard diver may execute twists and somersaults while he is airborne, but his centre of gravity will none the less follow a parabolic path and the equations describing its motion are simple. While the diver is still in contact with the springboard, one or two additional forces, due to action of board on feet come into play, but simple and important equations of motion for the centre of gravity may still be written.

Similarly, the gymnast or trampolinist, whether airborne or contacting equipment, the runner or cyclist rounding a curve or on the straight, and most other sporting actions, may be usefully studied in terms of the trajectory of the performer's centre of gravity and the forces *external* to the body. The simple equations which apply are well worth setting down, even if the study is later to investigate details of the motion of individual segments.

As examples, papers by Vaughan and Matravers (1977) on sprinting, and by Cavagna, Saibene, and Margaria (1963) on walking, bring out interesting points concerning the motion of the body's centre of gravity in locomotion.

Part-body models

It is often of interest to estimate what actions may be occurring in the main muscles and joints of the body during an activity and, if possible, to discover some secrets of successful athletic performance. In essence, the problem is to find the forces which are acting on individual segments, by separating each body segment from its neighbours, in concept, and revealing the joint and muscle forces which act within the limbs. The leg, for example, may be considered as three detached segments, foot, shank, and thigh. The action of major muscle groups, gastrocnemius, soleus, and so on, may be included in the model as tensile forces acting at the muscular points of attachment to bone. Such representation of muscles calls for anatomical knowledge and, of course, considerable simplification is necessary. If too many muscle actions are included, the number of unknown forces in the mathematical model soon becomes greater than the number of equations available, and the problem becomes indeterminate. Here again, the engineer's experience of judicious simplification of a system to attain a solution can well be applied. The assumptions made must be properly understood by anyone studying the results of such force calculations on the human body, and a high degree of accuracy cannot be expected. We should note that, whilst numerical estimates of force are useful, it is also important to exploit such mathematical modelling of internal actions to understand the nature of force transmission in the body. The importance of such studies in the understanding of sports injuries will be obvious. An interesting introduction to this topic can be found in Alexander and Vernon's (1975) paper.

Equipment design

The research and development work being carried out by sports equipment manufacturers is not usually available for general reading. As noted in the section on skiing in this chapter, some technical details may be made public for advertising purposes; new materials, modified shapes and styles, and improved internal structures are explained in some detail for the interested purchaser.

Many improvements are promoted by the challenge of international competitive sport. Designers and manufacturers work in liaison with top level competitors, so that design modification is a mixture of engineering skill and sensitive field assessment. Advances so made are often passed on quickly to the general public and competition between manufacturers is keen.

The canoeist, for example, has, over the last 20 years, seen many new slalom canoe designs appear on the market. Many of these were first proved successful in high-grade slalom competition, and prototypes were soon put into general production. Modification in hull shape seems to have been more a matter of canoeing experience and inspiration, than of research in hydrodynamics, and no less successful for that. Trends have been toward a flatter elliptical cross-section, a saucer-like underwater form for rapid turning, and a long pointed bow and stern riding clear of the water, except in turbulent conditions. Changes have had to be made within the constraints on hull shape imposed by competition regulations. Construction has for many years been in the durable and easily repaired glass-fibre reinforced plastics; canoes are moulded in two halves and joined at the gunwhale line, a line of weakness in even the best models. Perhaps the next wave of improvement in canoes will come with the newer technique of 'blown plastic' manufacture. A canoe of this type is truly a one-piece shell, which can be hammered, kicked, dropped from roof racks, and battered in surf, yet remain virtually unscathed.

All sports equipment design must rely on subjective assessment by the discerning user and the design problem often seems so complex that a more analytical approach is forbiddingly difficult. None the less, engineering expertise is valuable at the research as well as at the manufacturing stage. In Bleustein (1970), for instance, papers will be found on optimal design of an archery bow and the stresses in the strings and frames of tennis rackets. It seems certain that the coming decade will see a more fruitful marriage between scientific biomechanical analysis and subjective assessment in the design of sports equipment. The sport of skiing, more fully considered later, is benefiting from such liaisons and a fuller literature search will probably reveal similar progress in other areas of sport.

Man–equipment interaction

Ergonomics, the science of man at work, incorporates the study of human response to environmental demands and is concerned with interactions between man and machine. The term 'sports ergonomics' is little used, but sport is a form of human work and the interactions between the sportsman and his equipment are of real interest in biomechanics.

The simpler interactions occur when the surroundings remain relatively constant; the more complex interactions take place when there is continual change in the interactive forces. Thus, simpler cases are seen in the runner travelling at steady speed over a firm level track, the skier 'schussing' in a straight line down a constant gradient, or the cyclist pedalling at constant speed on the level. Instances of more complex interactions between man and surroundings are seen when the runner tackles a mountain route, the skier executes turns with varying speed and radius, and the cyclist faces hill-climb conditions.

The mechanics of the human body alone is difficult enough; analysis of man–equipment interactions will be even more troublesome. None the less, insight is being gained into this intriguing region. Consider the pole-vaulter. His body actions cause changes both in his own body configuration and in the curvature of the fibreglass vaulting pole. For informative first reading on the dynamics of these interacting systems, we turn once more to Bleustein (1970) for a paper on 'Computer modelling of pole vaulting'. A simple conceptual model leads to most interesting results. The model regards the pole as a light uniform rod with known flexural stiffness, whilst the vaulter is represented as a mass of variable moment of inertia and of variable centre of gravity position, relative to the handhold location on the pole. In the simulations, the actions taken by the athlete during the jump are known *a priori* and perfectly executed, presumably from film analysis of good performances on real poles. Once the governing equations are established, computer solutions provide for a range of conditions. Variations in pole stiffness, handhold height, and take-off technique are investigated, and a good deal of understanding gained with this apparently simple model of the activity. As with any mathematical model, the constraints embodied in the first model may be relaxed in later studies and a more realistic representation of the situation attempted. The price must be paid in more difficult mathematical formulations and longer computer programs.

In the same volume of research papers (Bleustein 1970), a much more elaborate man–machine simulation is presented. This is a computer simulation of bicycle dynamics and development of the cycle-rider model runs through 140 equations before reaching its final form. Computer runs were programmed to provide graphical representations of the position of cycle and rider during various manoeuvres, and these results were checked against film of real cycling tests.

Feedback control

Sports psychologists often refer to the concept of 'feedback', implying that the senses receive information monitoring the results of actions taken and the performer then utilizes this information to modify future actions. Such feeding back of data to assist control seems universal in living organisms, and in sport the concept is obviously most relevant. The experimental psychologist does not appear to venture into mathematical models of feedback, although he builds up a picture of probable feedback pathways utilized by the nervous and muscular systems.

In sports biomechanics the concept of feedback must be seen as a natural extension of the study of man–equipment interaction, albeit a difficult one. Milsum (1966) opens the door to this field of human performance study. Once again, it is the establishment of a mathematical model of the process of feedback control which gives fundamental understanding of the interactions between elements of the system. Research publications in this area are few in number, though an example from skiing is cited in the next section.

Descriptive mechanics or kinesiology

The student of physical education is usually introduced to biomechanics by a descriptive presentation of essential concepts, such as force, static equilibrium, momentum, work, and energy. Such technical terms from mechanics are being increasingly used among teachers and performers, in sports instruction manuals, and by sports commentators. Popular mechanics seems to be regarded as common knowledge. Unfortunately, while these technical concepts can be most useful, the danger is that terms become loosely used in general conversation and lose their accuracy and effect. Momentum, energy, and other such terms can easily become 'OK words' which merely lend a technical air to the proceedings.

Ideally, kinesiology or descriptive mechanics of movement, should aid clear thinking on the principles of human motion, force production, balance, and effective co-ordination. Of the available texts, those of Dyson (1977), Hopper (1973), and Kelley (1971) should give much food for thought to sportsmen and teachers of physical education in all areas.

Statistical studies

Some work on human performance, particularly in child development and the effects of sports training, are concerned with groups of subjects and the factors are analysed statistically. Sometimes the study requires the measurement of biomechanical variables, such as running speed, height of jump, force applied in a strength test, or angles of limb segments during a filmed activity. In such cases the work has a biomechanical element. Although statistical analysis is less searching than detailed mathematical modelling of the activity in question, with many variable factors under consideration, statistical methods may provide the only means of analysing the results.

An example of this type of study is a paper by Bloomfield, Elliott, and Davies (1979) describing film analysis of kicking for 56 boys, aged between 2 and 12 years. Several kinematic factors, approach speed, leg segment angles, and angular velocities, were measured from the cinematographic record. Means and standard deviations of these variables were calculated for six sub-groups. These latter were identified by certain characteristics of their kicking action, a general progression in age and kicking skill being seen through the groups. Other biomechanical research, involving more factors, has called for the use of analysis of variance and factor analysis techniques.

Physiological studies

Electromyography, in which small voltages generated in the tissue by active muscle give an indication of the presence and order of magnitude of a muscular action, is a widely used technique in biomechanical studies. It is somewhat contentious whether electromyographic measuring devices can be employed to estimate muscle-tension force, but some claims in this direction have been made.

A second area concerns links between exercise physiology and biomechanics. Common ground exists in that both disciplines are concerned with the measurement of energy, work, and power. The physiologist deals more with biomechanical aspects of energy release and its availability to the body. In biomechanics, we can evaluate the kinetic and potential energies of body segments in motion during a dynamic analysis and show how much of the available energy is required for these actions. Biomechanics also deals with energy required to overcome external resistances, whether of the air, as in cycling, or of water, as in swimming. Studies bridging the gap between biomechanics and physiology are not common, and there is much scope for further liaison between the two disciplines. An interesting work on human locomotion is provided by Margaria *et al.* (1963).

Application of biomechanics to skiing

The foregoing subsections cite only a small sample of biomechanical papers covering a handful of sports. In this section we examine one sport in a little more detail. Skiing provides many examples of the application of biomechanics, as defined at the beginning of this chapter. Most of the areas listed in Table 6.1 are represented in the skiing literature and, with increasing participation in the sport, technical matters must be considered not only by the instructor, but also by the recreational skier.

Useful initial material for study will be found in the collection of papers by Bleustein (1970). Ski research papers appear under the following titles:

(a) 'On the mechanics of skis'.
(b) 'The mechanics of snow–ski interaction during a carved turn'.
(c) 'Analytical studies of the biomechanics of contemporary ski bindings'.
(d) 'Remarks on the dynamic performance of ski release bindings'.
(e) 'The dynamic torsional response of the human leg, relative to skiing injuries'.

Papers (a) and (b) deal primarily with the engineering properties of skis in bending and torsion; there has been rapid advance in recent years in the design and construction of skis. A good deal of the research has been carried out by ski manufacturers in Europe and America, but their laboratory reports may not be easily obtained. Technical advances in ski design have been prompted by the need for high-grade equipment for international slalom and downhill racing. Prototype designs are tested by top performers under training and race conditions, and from their subjective assessments the design engineer attempts to modify the ski's response by changes in construction. The internal form of a modern ski is usually a carefully planned structure of hollow cells and laminations, providing high strength with light-weight, a desired pattern of bending stiffness along the ski, and a degree of damping to the bending and twisting vibrations which cause the ski to 'chatter' at high speed. The full engineering details may not be of interest to most skiers, but certain aspects of the construction and properties of a ski are now quoted in suppliers' catalogues.

Papers (c), (d), and (e) are more concerned with safety aspects of skiing. As with the skis themselves, bindings, linking the boot to the ski, have benefited from many design improvements over the last decade. The aim has been to reduce ski injuries. Modern bindings should release the boot and leg in all manner of forward, sideways, and twisting falls and may be accurately set for higher release loads as the skier becomes more competent and travels faster. These three papers illustrate three of the problems of binding design.

Paper (c) deals with laboratory tests on the release of bindings with slowly applied forces. Such experiments provide essential data on the loads applied to the leg during a fall and adjustments in release force which are consistent with safety.

Paper (d) examines the response of bindings to vibration, simulating the effects of ski-running over uneven snow and conditions which sometimes cause unwanted release of bindings.

In paper (e) the twisting actions on the leg during skiing are discussed, especially those situations where torsional fracture of the tibia may occur.

Since the publication of these papers in 1970, much more work has been done on ski performance and safety. An important series of papers is associated with the Mechanical Engineering Laboratories of the Universities of California and Standford. We consider here three of the more recent contributions to this continuing work to illustrate the techniques employed in this area of investigation.

(1) 'A preliminary analysis of ski release binding dynamic properties' (Mote and Hull 1976) presents a mathematical model of a ski binding, incorporating inertial and torsional–elastic properties of the leg–boot unit, friction in the binding, and rotational inertia of the ski. A laboratory rig consisting of ski, binding, boot, and a vertical shaft to represent the tibia, was constructed and three commercial bindings were tested, the torque–rotation characteristics providing the main experimental results. The authors make the significant remark that the manufacturers showed no consensus regarding the desirable torque–rotation behaviour of a binding. The laboratory rig was instrumented with strain gauges to measure the torque in the vertical 'tibial' shaft and a potentiometer to pick off the shaft rotation. Suitable data processors provided direct plots of torque against rotation as the tests proceeded.

Alongside the experimental results, the mathematical model is developed. The equations of motion are solved and theoretical plots of torque versus rotation are compared with those obtained experimentally. Similarity of form in these two sets of results confirms that the mathematical model is a good theoretical representation of the binding test rig, and justifies the assumptions and simplifications introduced to make the mathematics manageable. It is then possible to use the equations of the model to investigate the effects of sudden impulsive loads applied to the system, an effect difficult to achieve experimentally. Impulse loading is important because it is frequently the cause of premature release of the binding, a dangerous occurrence at high speed. The mathematical formulation commences with a second-order differential equation of motion and incorporates the non-linear behaviour of the binding due to friction. One of the simplifying assumptions in the published work is that the musculature of the leg has no resisting effect on the torsion of the leg. This, and other assumptions in the preliminary study, are to be relaxed in later work. As with all mathematical modelling, the model is not only a means for providing accurate numerical data; it shows also the dynamic interactions between the elements of a system and clarifies its essential behaviour.

(2) In 'A dynamic non-linear finite element model of the human leg' Hight, Piziali and Nagel (1979) report on the development of a mathematical model of the whole-leg action in skiing. The model accommodates large three-dimensional displacements and rotations and the non-linear stiffness of the knee joint. Starting with the concept of the segmental model, motion of the lower limb is first thought of as displacement of a simple hinged mechanism in the vertical plane. This basic form is then extended to represent the leg more realistically and a five-segment model, with soft non-linear springs linking elastically deformable segments, is set out. Development of the governing equations forms a major part of the paper, and energy methods from engineering structural dynamics are employed for the solution.

Computer solutions of the mathematical model are obtained for several conditions of the system. The most interesting uses input loadings to the leg which are derived from direct force measurements at the binding during aggressive downhill parallel skiing. Hight and his colleagues conclude their paper with computed values of stress concentration across the tibial cross-section, finding that peak tensile stresses in the ski tests are close to the yield stress for bone at certain points. The authors, having made an important contribution to modelling the dynamic response of the human, await experimental measurements of damping and active muscle forces in the leg for further development of their work.

(3) Finally, in this sample of ski-safety research papers, comes Hull and Mote's (1980) 'Leg loading in snow skiing: computer analyses'. This paper is in the series of publications by the same authors at the University of California Mechanical Engineering Laboratories. Earlier work reported the development of strain-gauge force transducers, located in a ski under the toe and heel of the boot and each capable of measuring three components of force and three force-moment components. Thus, the force systems at toe and heel were completely specified and the location of the transducers within the ski allowed normal boot positioning in the binding. A telemetry system, using pulse-code modulation, was carried in a small backpack and transmitted the fluctuating force and moment values to a receiver up to 3 km away during downhill skiing in four styles. These ski-turn techniques, the snow-plough, the stem-christie, the slow parallel, and the fast parallel, repre-

sented the main stages of expertise in skiing. The 1980 paper deals with the analysis of the complex force–time records obtained in these earlier field trials. The force data are analysed in terms of their frequency structure by power spectrum techniques and correlations between pairs of forces and moments are also obtained. The authors conclude that muscular contraction in the leg influences the release properties of the binding and that, ideally, binding release should be sensitive to muscular activity. Comment is also made that forward twisting falls are frequent in skiing and that correlation between forward bending and twisting loads on the leg is to be expected on such occasions. It is expected that continuation of the research will produce more field data on actual skiing falls and realistic analysis of the leg loading in the extremely short period of fall and binding release will be possible. Laboratory development of an electronic binding is mentioned and it seems probable that a commercial version may appear in the near future.

The eight ski research papers outlined here range over many technical topics and their links with the areas of sports biomechanics activity 3, 4 and 6–8 as listed in Table 6.1 will be apparent. To many students of biomechanics, whose main interest is in sports science or physical education, such papers may seem too biased toward engineering methods, the motion of the human body itself being inadequately represented. To redress the balance, ski publications in some other areas of biomechanical activity must be mentioned.

Sodeyama, Miura, Kitamura, and Matsui (1976) have studied the displacement of a skier's centre of gravity during a parallel ski turn, using two cameras to record the motion and to provide displacement data on the body segments. From these data the three-dimensional trajectory of the centre of gravity was computed. This is essentially a kinematic study, but the authors comment upon the force actions associated with the recorded motion, without calculating numerical values. Such observations are kinesiological in nature. Biomechanics areas 2, 5, and 10 of Table 6.1 are, therefore, represented.

Force measurement applying to whole-body motion is reported by Watanabe and Ohtsuki (1977) in their 'Postural changes and aerodynamic forces in Alpine skiing', whilst an application of feedback control theory will be found in 'A control system's approach to ski turn analysis' (Morawski 1973). These papers illustrate areas 3 and 9 as listed in Table 6.1.

Broader issues, such as methods of ski instruction, studies of ski technique, and the occurrence of ski injuries are covered by United States University theses and dissertations, official national ski teaching manuals and, in the case of European work, by a bibliography due to Aubert (1974). The reader delving into biomechanical sources will be well served if he has a firm grasp of the principles of mechanics. Particularly in the kinesiological or 'descriptive mechanics' area, basic principles may be somewhat carelessly used in explaining human performance. In one skiing text, Newton's Third Law of Motion is called in to support an argument which is, in fact, an application of a quite different theorem, the Principle of Moments; and, elsewhere, momentum (mass × velocity) is deemed to be the same as force (mass × acceleration). Despite such confusion, good descriptive mechanics can be most helpful in elucidating the principles on which skilled action depends (Table 6.1, area 10).

Finally, in this glance at the skiing literature, the equipment suppliers' catalogues must be considered. A typical 1980 catalogue provides descriptive and diagrammatic information on the main ski types – 'compact', 'mid-length', and 'standard' – and gives details of their internal structures, describing foam, hexagonal cell, and laminated cores, with built-in vibration absorbing materials and a range of flexural properties suitable for specific snow conditions and skiing techniques. Bindings and boots are similarly described in terms of their technical performance and it must be supposed that a proportion of readers and purchasers will understand this material. Manufacturers naturally wish to show how much technical development has taken place and even recreational skiers are becoming increasingly serious about the equipment they buy, and its influence on their performance. Technical interest will surely continue to grow with increasing participation in the sport (Table 6.1, areas 7 and 8).

References

Alexander, R. M. and Vernon, A. (1975). The dimensions of knee and ankle muscles and the forces they exert. *J. Hum. Movt. Stud.* **3**, 115–23.

Aubert, H. (1974). *Skiing: an international preliminary bibliography 1968–73*. Norges Inrettshogskole. Oslo.

Bleustein, J. L. (ed.) (1970). *Mechanics and sport.* Am. Soc. Mech. Engrs, New York.

Bloomfield, J. Elliott, B. C. and Davies, C. M. (1979). Development of the soccer kick: a cinematographical analysis. *J. Hum. Movt. Stud.* **5**, 152–9.

Braune, W. and Fischer, O. (1889). Centre of gravity of the human body as related to the equipment of German infantry. [In German] *Treatises of the mathematical physics class of the Royal Academy of Sciences of Saxony*, 7.

Cavagna, G. A. Saibene, F. P. and Margaria, R. (1963). External work in walking. *J. app;. Physiol.* **18**, 1–9.

Dempster, W. T. (1955). Space requirements of the seated operator. *WADC Tech. Rep.* No. 55–159. Wright-Patterson Air Force Base, Ohio.

Dyson, G. H. G. (1977). *The mechanics of athletics.* Hodder & Stoughton, London.

Grieve, D. W. (1968). Gait patterns and the speed of walking. *Biomed. Engng.* **3**, 119.

Hanavan, E. P. (1964). A mathematical model of the human body. *WADC Tech. Rep.* TR64-102. Wright-Patterson Air Force Base, Ohio.

Hatze, H. (1977). A complete set of control equations for the human musculo-skeletal system. *J. Biomech.* **10**, 799–805.

Hight, T. K., Piziali, R. H. and Nagel, D. A. (1979). A dynamic non-linear finite-element model of the human leg. *Trans. Am. Soc. Mech. Engrs.* **101**, 176–84.

Hopper, B. J. (1973). *Biomechanics of human motion.* Crosby, Lockwood, Staples, London.

Hull, M. L. and Mote, C. D. (1980). Leg loading in snow skiing: computer analyses. *J. Biomech.* **13**, 481–91.

Hull, M. L. and Mote, C. D. (1978). Analysis of leg loading in snow skiing. *J. Dynam. Syst., Measurement and Control.* **100**, 177–86.

Kelley, D. L. (1971). *Kinesiology*. Prentice Hall, New Jersey.

Lees, A. G. (1980). An optimised film analysis method based on finite difference techniques. *J. Hum. Movt. Stud.* **6**, 165–80.

Margaria, R., Cerretelli, P., Aghemo, P. and Sassi, G. (1963). Energy cost of running. *J. appl. Physiol.* **18**, 367–70.

Milsum, J. H. (1966). *Biological control systems analysis.* McGraw Hill, London.

Morawski, J. M. (1973). Control systems approach to ski turn analysis. *J. Biomech.* **6**, 267–75.

Mote, C. D. and Hull, M. L. (1976). A preliminary analysis of ski release binding dynamic properties. *J. Dynam. Syst., Measurement and Control.* **98**, 1–8.

Plagenhoef, S. (1971). *Patterns of human motion.* Prentice Hall, New Jersey.

Santschi, W. R., Dubois, J. and Omoto, C. (1963). Moments of inertia and centres of gravity of the living human body. *AMLR Tech. Doc. Rep.* 63–36. Wright-Patterson Air Force Base, Ohio.

Sodeyama, H., Miura, M., Kitamura, K. and Matsui, H. (1975). Study of the displacement of a skier's centre of gravity during a ski turn. In *Biomechanics,* (ed.) P. V. Komi, Vol. V(B). University Park Press, Pennsylvania.

Smith, A. J. (1972). A study of the forces on the body in athletic activities, with particular reference to jumping. Ph.D. Thesis, University of Leeds.

Vaughan, C. L. and Matravers, D. R. (1977). A biomechanical model of the sprinter. *J. Hum. Movt. Stud.* **3**, 207–13.

Watanabe, K. and Ohtsuki, T. (1977). Postural changes and aerodynamic forces in Alpine skiing. *Ergonomics.* **20**, 121–32.

Whitsett, C. E. (1963). Some dynamic response characteristics of weightless man. *AMRL Tech. Doc. Rep.* 63–18. Wright-Patterson Air Force Base, Ohio.

Winter, D. A., Sidwall, H. G. and Hobson, D. A. (1974). Measurement and reduction of noise in kinematics of locomotion. *J. Biomech.* **7**, 157–9.

7 Athletic achievement – trends and limits

B. B. LLOYD

In a Presidential Address to the British Association (Lloyd 1966) the thesis was set out that for a runner to obtain kinetic energy to cover the ground horizontally, his body uses metabolic energy from two sources: an oxygen-independent store in the active muscles, and a supply derived from the oxidation of glycogen by oxygen brought to the muscles from the air by respiration and circulation. The argument was at that time summarized in the equation.

$$S(1 - e^{-gt}) + (R - A)(t - \Delta t) = \alpha\, mv^2/2 + By, \qquad (7.1)$$

in which the availability of the store S is governed by the rate constant g, the oxygen-dependent rate of energy supply R is used to the extent of A for non-running metabolism and delayed for a small initial interval Δt, and α is a factor relating metabolic energy to the kinetic energy of the body $mv^2/2$. B (with the value 64.8) is the number of metabolic calories needed to transport a standard runner (72 kg) over one metre, embodying the fundamental concept, fully discussed previously (Lloyd 1966), that this metabolic energy expenditure is, air resistance apart, independent of the runner's speed.

Subsequently, a term $C\int_0^t v^3 \mathrm{d}t$ was introduced to represent the metabolic energy used in overcoming air resistance (Lloyd 1967), and later it was concluded (Lloyd and Moran 1966) that the efficiency E of conversion of metabolic energy into kinetic energy and work against air drag was probably nearer 50 per cent than 25 per cent, and that Δt, the delay in the use of R, was approximately zero. The equation thus took the form

$$y = S(1 - e^{-gt})/B + (R - A)t/B - \alpha mv^2/(2B) - C\int_0^t v^3 \mathrm{d}t/B. \qquad (7.2)$$

These conclusions followed the use of an analogue computer to represent the modified equation and to yield graphs of distance and velocity against time. Subsequently the equation was solved numerically on a digital computer, so that it became possible (Lloyd 1967) to calculate the effects of altitude by introducing the factors p multiplying R and q multiplying C. These enabled plausible predictions to be made of results at the Mexico City Olympics (Anonymous 1968), which were quite well borne out in practice (Lloyd 1969), except those for swimming, to which reference is made later.

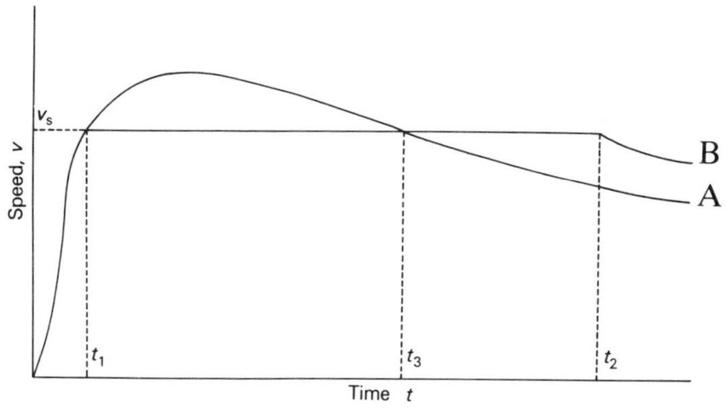

Fig. 7.1. Time–velocity profiles of a flat-out run A and a run B with steady (coasting) speed v_s. The time taken from start to reach v_s is t_1, and the times at which v_s can no longer be maintained are t_3 and t_2 on the flat-out and steady-speed runs respectively. (Lloyd and Zacks 1972.)

The next advances were to incorporate an incomplete theory of the extra power needed to run on a circular track (Lloyd 1969), and to show (Lloyd and Zacks 1972) that in races longer than 400 m it is profitable not to run flat-out – as is implied by the original equation – but to accelerate to a critical coasting speed, to maintain this to a breaking point, and then to run flat-out while decelerating towards the tape (Fig. 7.1). The effects of coasting speed on the time for a given race are shown in Fig. 7.2 for the mile to the 800 m, and in Fig. 7.3 for the 800 m to the 400 m, the longest race for which no optimal coasting speed is discernible, which implies that for races of 400 m or less running flat-out yields the shortest times. The differences between flat-out and optimized running patterns above 400 m are small but important, estimated to be about 6 m for the 800 m race, 12 m for the 1500 m, 16 m for the 5000 m, and 17 m for the 10 000 m event and beyond. It was argued (Lloyd 1969) that curvature in effect increased weight or the factor B in eqn (7.1) by a factor $1 + v^4/(2G^2\varrho^2)$, in which v is speed, G the acceleration due to gravity, and ϱ the radius of curvature. The corrections predicted by this factor are rather smaller than those for optimization, ranging for a track 45 m in radius from 3.6 m for the 200 m event through about 5 m for the 400 and 800 m to 6 m for the 1500 m, 14 m for the 5000 and 24 m for the 10 000 m event, increasing thereafter in rough proportion to distance; the curvature corrections for women are about 2/3 those for men. To convert an optimized performance on a part-straight, part-circular track to the equivalent run flat-out on a straight track – as represented by the equation – the optimization correction has to be subtracted from the real distance and the curvature correction added, and for most purposes in this paper actual distances have been so modified.

In 1965 and 1966 it was suggested that the linearity of the time–distance

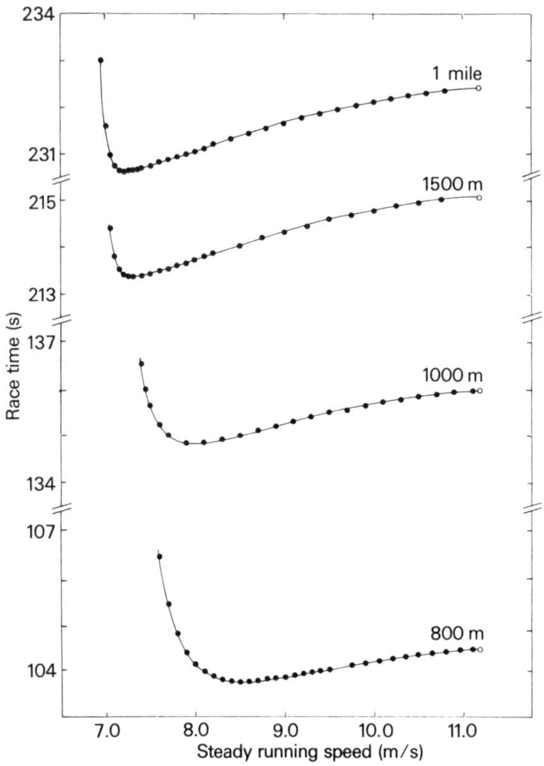

Fig. 7.2. Relation between race times and coasting speed v_s as determined by computer analysis, for distances of 800 m, 1000 m, 1500 m, and 1 mile; open circles denote flat-out runs. (Lloyd and Zacks 1972.)

plots for the six ranges covering 50 yd to 623 miles (45 m to 1000 km) (Fig. 7.4) implied a separate store-rate couple for each range. It now seems more satisfactory to regard the apparently real discontinuities between the ranges as largely due to the frequency with which certain races are run, and to represent the decline in the rate of energy supply exhibited in longer races by means of a second exponential term. Thus in the equation

$$R = R_i + hU, \tag{7.3}$$

R represents the total rate of oxygen-supported energy used and R_i the component indefinitely available for the longest runs when U is exhausted, hU representing an oxygen-dependent contribution from a source which diminishes with time at a rate governed by the constant h. The metabolic energy yielded over time t is thus

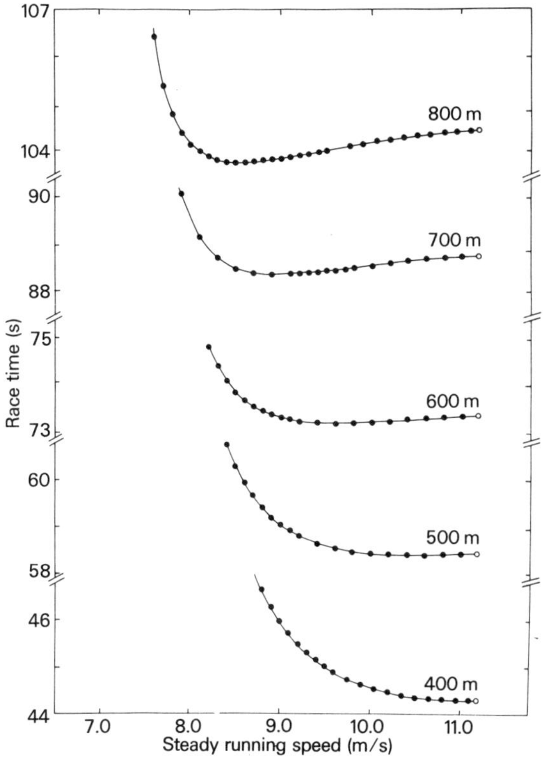

Fig. 7.3. Relation between race times and coasting speed v_s as determined by computer analysis, for distances of 400, 500, 600, 700, and 800 m; open circles denote flat-out runs. (Lloyd and Zacks 1972.)

$$\int_0^t R\mathrm{d}t = R_i t + U(1 - e^{-ht}) \tag{7.4}$$

Like the exponential term in eqn (7.1) that in eqn (7.4) relates to flat-out running in which the ever-diminishing product hU is maximized by sufficient effort. Runners do not necessarily run like this, but, as with the first exponential relating to short-term optimizations, probably run to optimize energy use, and to produce time–distance plots for longer races that are not very different from those predicted by eqn (7.4).

An alternative but mathematically equivalent formulation to eqn (7.3) is to posit that

$$R = R_i + R_0 e^{-ht} . \tag{7.5}$$

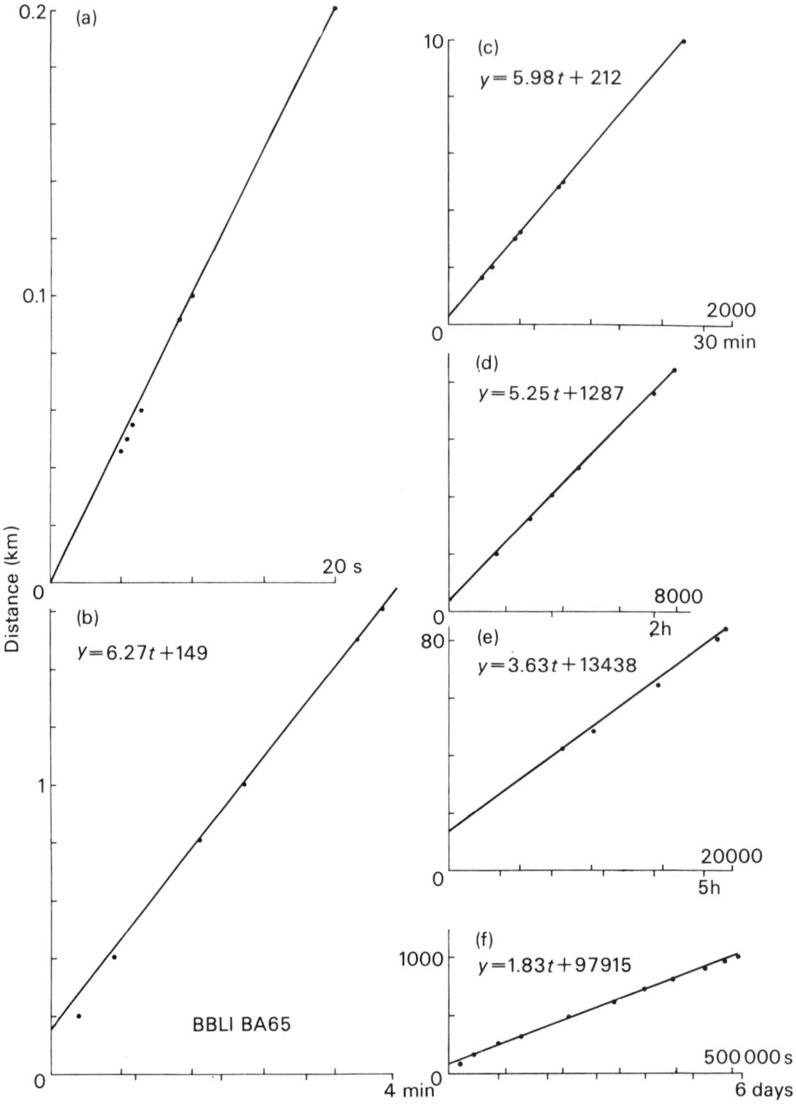

Fig. 7.4. Records for male runners, 50 yd to 623 miles, on 26 August, 1965. Distance (km) plotted against time (s) on linear scales. Equations are calculated in terms of metres for lines through fastest points and correspond with the equation,

$$y = S/B + t(R - A)/B.$$

Intercepts are related to energy stores, slopes to rates of energy supply. Slopes are visually comparable. (Lloyd 1966.)

where R_0 is an initial rate component which declines exponentially, and which gives the total oxygen-supported energy over time t as

$$\int_0^t R\mathrm{d}T = R_i t + R_0(1 - \mathrm{e}^{-ht})/h, \qquad (7.6)$$

where R_0 equals hU of eqn (7.3).

Equation (7.1) needs considerable amplification to include these ideas, and in its full form may be written

$$S(1 - \mathrm{e}^{-gt}) + pU(1 - \mathrm{e}^{-ht}) + pR_i t$$
$$= \alpha\, mv^2/(2E) + qC'a \int_0^t v^3\mathrm{d}t/E + bmy\,(1 + v^4/(2G^2\varrho^2)), \qquad (7.7)$$

where R_i has for simplicity already had A (non-running power) subtracted, B has been replaced by bm (b being cal/kg body mass m per metre run), and E being the efficiency of conversion of metabolic into external work; α (0.2389) converts joules into calories; p is a factor (1 at sea level) to allow for reduced oxygen supply at high altitude, q is less than 1 when air density is reduced as at altitiude, and C', as opposed to C, takes account of cross-sectional area a and the external mechanical work (in calories) needed to overcome air resistance.

Manipulation of eqn (7.7) yields distance y for a flat-out run as a function of t, velocity, and curvature:

$$y = S(1 - \mathrm{e}^{-gt})/(bm) + pU(1 - \mathrm{e}^{-ht})/(bm) + p\,R_i t/(bm)$$
$$- \alpha\, v^2/(2bE) - qC'a \int_0^t v^3\mathrm{d}t/(bmE) - yv^4/(2G^2\varrho^2)\ ; \qquad (7.8)$$

i.e. distance is promoted by the first store, the second store, and the steady rate, and is reduced for kinetic energy, air resistance, and curvature.

We can lighten further discussion by omitting the curvature term (setting ϱ at ∞) and omitting the altitude factors p and q, so that

$$y = S(1 - \mathrm{e}^{-gt})/(bm) + U(1 - \mathrm{e}^{-ht})/(bm) + R_i t/(bm)$$
$$- \alpha v^2/(2bE) - C'a \int_0^t v^3\mathrm{d}t/(bmE). \qquad (7.9)$$

Furthermore, size seems of little significance in running, and it is reasonable to assume that S, U, and R are all proportional to m, and to replace $S/(bm)$, $U/(bm)$ and $R_i/(bm)$ by s, u, and r. Over the narrow range of sizes of adult men it is also reasonable, though perhaps not exact, to regard a as proportional to m and to replace $C'a/(bm)$ with c, giving

$$y = s(1 - e^{-gt}) + u(1 - e^{-ht}) + rt$$
$$- kv^2/E - c \int_0^t v^3 dt/E, \qquad (7.10)$$

in which each term represents a distance; $k = a/2b = 0.133\ s^2/m$ and b is 0.9 cal/kg body mass/horizontal metre, bm equalling B of eqn (7.1); c has been estimated by Pugh (1971) and by Hill (1928), whose results for a man of cross-sectional area 0.5 m^2 give $c = 0.0010125\ s^2/m^2$. For a man of 72 kg and cross-sectional area 0.5 m^2 eqn (7.9) finally yields

$$y = s(1 - e^{-gt}) + u(1 - e^{-ht}) + rt$$
$$- 0.133\ v^2/E - 0.0010125 \int_0^t v^3 dt/E. \qquad (7.11)$$

It is worthwhile reminding ourselves at this point that the equation, in which each term is a distance, purports to represent the time–distance relationship of a flat-out runner, and, when appropriate adjustments are made, the time–distance relations of optimally run races or speed trials extending from very short to very long distances. The equation cannot be solved by algebraic methods, but if values of the parameters are given it is possible to run the equation on an analogue or digital computer, and to produce values of distance, velocity, energy, etc., at any value of t.

The problem is, however, to obtain values of the parameters from a set of y, t data such as the world records of a selected year. This can be approached graphically, and in 1965 using the current world records for the curtailed eqn (7.1) it was deduced that $S/B = 164$ m, $g = 0.0397\ s^{-1}$, and $(R - A)/B = 6.27$ m/s. Later, with an analogue computer, the air-resistance term was incorporated (Lloyd and Moran 1966) and a good fit was obtained for the data up to 1500 m with $S/B = 212$, $g = 0.050$, $(R - A) = 6.847$, $\Delta t =$ O, and $E = 0.5$.

The subject was taken further (Zacks 1971) using a digital computer to obtain values of the parameters by an iterative optimizing procedure incorporating a Runge–Kutta numerical solution of the equation, the sum of the squares of the residuals (distance predicted–distance run) being minimized. Zacks (1971) obtained nine sets of parameters for the world records for men in various years up to 1970, and concluded, on the assumption that efficiency was 50 per cent, both for accelerating the body and for overcoming drag, that S/B was substantially constant, that g had increased by perhaps 10 per cent since 1870, and that $(R - A)/B$, the oxygen dependent energy supply, had increased by about 20 per cent.

Recently the parameters of eqn (7.11) were obtained by minimizing the sums of the squared residuals $(Y\text{-}y)/y$, y being distance run, mainly with world records for men. There was some difficulty in getting the program to converge in reasonable time with all parameters being allowed to move freely, but convergence was achieved with 13 records for 1980 ranging from 60 yards 100 miles, giving reasonable values for s, g, u, h, and r, but high values for efficiency. In fact, the efficiency was allowed to vary independently for the acceleration term and the drag term, resulting in E_a at 0.81 and E_d at 0.93. These figures are not inconsistent with the work of Cavagna and Kaneko (1977) or with some of the results of Pugh (1971), and imply some elastic storage of energy in tendon or contracted muscle. It was, therefore, decided to obtain a set of parameters from records from 60 yards to 100 miles for 1980, 65 and 52 with E fixed, for acceleration and for drag, at 0.75, and another set with $E = 0.5$. The fit was about twice as good (Σ res^2 half as big) with $E = 0.75$ as with $E = 0.5$, and the values for u and h (the long-term store) were consistent with the notion, indicated by some earlier iterations, that u and h do not change from year to year. These parameters (E, u, and h) were then fixed for all the years examined at the values given by the 1980 data, and values for parameters s, g, and r found for all the years. This showed that s, if anything, appeared to decrease with time as the years rolled on, which is physiologically highly improbable as it implies B increasing or S decreasing or both, so s was fixed for all sets of data at the 1980 value, and a final set of iterations performed with $s = 215.1$, $z = 51\ 250$, $h = 0.0000737$ gives the results for g and r plotted in Fig. 7.5. The residuals are in general <1 per cent.

The trends in Fig. 7.5 are interesting: g, the rate constant governing the use of s, the small store (sometimes equated with the 'oxygen debt') seems to have increased fairly steadily until 1939 and since then to have been constant, whereas r, the indefinitely available oxygen-using energy supply, has increased fairly steadily since 1874 and linearly since 1939. The implications may be that the set of parameters operating in AD 2000 will be $s = 215.2$, $g = 0.04042$, $u = 51\ 250$, $h = 0.0000737$, $r = 3.0627$, and $E = 0.75$. Table 7.1 gives some of the results generated by these parameters, which are also entered on Fig. 7.6, for comparison with actual records since the 1860s.

The trends in g and r are interesting and encourage some speculation: g looks as if it may be at the top end of a sigmoid expansion, whereas r may be on the quasilinear part, and liable to turn over into a flat top at any time. It may be assumed that g is biochemical and intracellular in nature, and possible not very amenable to training, whereas r is dominated by the

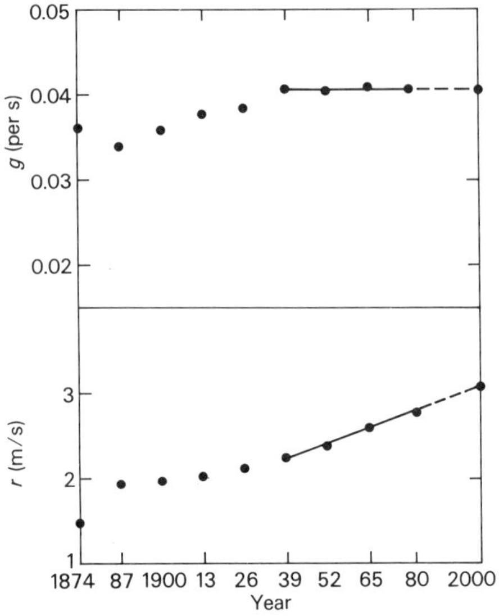

Fig. 7.5. Parameters g and r of eqn 7.11 plotted against calendar year. Other parameters are fixed. Points for the year 2000 were obtained by linear extrapolation.

carriage of oxygen respiration and circulation, both of which are amenable to training.

The nature of the long-term store u is of interest. In distance units it is 51 250 m, 20 per cent longer than the marathon, and corresponding fairly closely with the glycogen stores of the active muscles. As it gets used up the

Table 7.1 *Extrapolations of world records for men to the year 2000*

Distance (m)	Actual time 1980	Extrapolated time 2000
100	9.95 s	9.82 s
200	19.72 (at alt.)	19.63
400	43.86 (at alt.)	42.60
800	1:42.4	1:38.8
1500	3:31.4	3:25.9
1609.35 (mile)	3:48.8	3:42.7
3000	7:32.1	7:20.7
5000	13:08.4	12:36.9
10 000	27:22.3	26: 3.8
Marathon 42 195	2 h 8:34	2 h 2:21
160 935 (100 miles)	11 h 30:51	10 h 38:9
1 hour	20 944 m	21 988 m

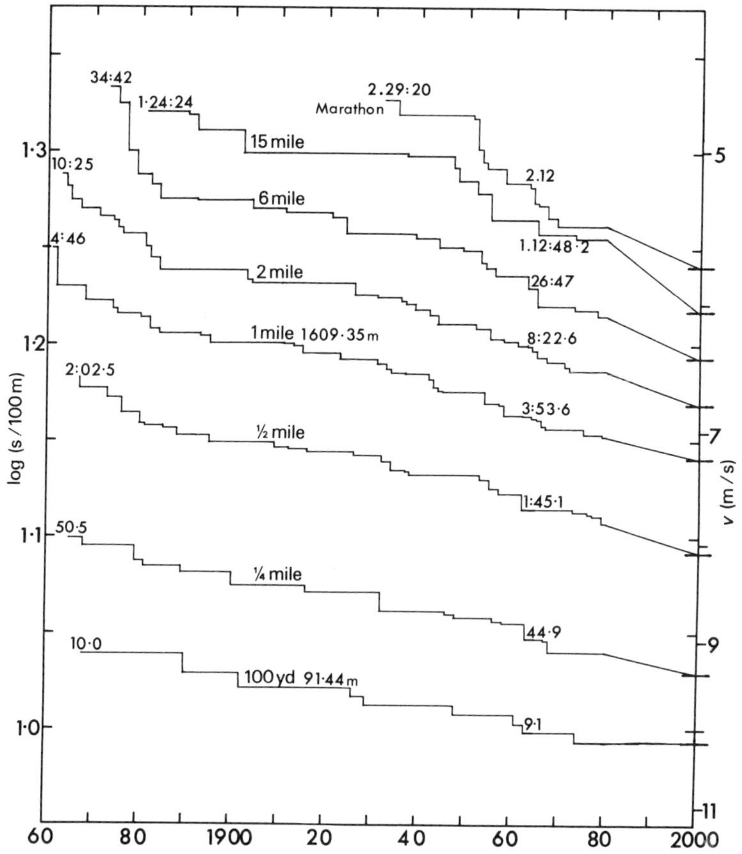

Fig. 7.6. Time trends in male running records, 1861–1965–1980–2000. Log of average time (in s) taken to run 100 m is plotted against calendar year. Corresponding velocity in m/s on a logarithmic scale is shown on the right-hand ordinate. Times of first and 1965 records are written against stepped line for each race. Points for the year 2000 are conjectural.

maximum rate of oxygen usage seems to fall, and the mechanism of this is of great interest.

Women present a somewhat similar picture, with an even greater rate of improvement. Some of the parameters that do not vary consistently with time are probably genuinely, though not very greatly, different from those of men, and the time-dependent parameters are given in Table 7.2. The values obtained by linear extrapolation to AD 2000 have been used in the equation to give the time–distance values in Table 7.3.

Some data for skating from Olympic record results are summarized in Fig. 7.7–7.9. The first point emerging from the time–distance plots is the extreme linearity for men over the range 1500–10 000 m and for women over

Table 7.2 *Parameters of the equation of motion (eqn 7.10) of women over the years,* $s = 251.2$ m, $E = 0.75$, $n =$ 51 250 m, and $h = 0.00006326$

AD	g (per s)	r (m/s)
1980	0.02771	2.383
1965	0.02877	1.893
1952	0.02924	1.405
1939	0.02984	1.239
1926	0.02646	0.808

the range of 1000–3000 m, so that the store-rate hypothesis seems to apply. The intercept is clearly defined and apparently invariant over time for men at 183 m and women at 111 m, representing the distance supported by the short-term store, which, according to the plot for women, cannot be completely spent in the first 500 m. The slope represents the rate at which energy can be supplied, presumably by oxygen-using processes, and these slopes are plotted against calendar year in Fig. 7.9. The men's slope might well reach 12.25 by AD 2000, but where the women will be is debatable. In the 1980 Olympics the women skated about as fast as the men in the 1960 Olympics.

Figure 7.10 shows that in 1980, at distances of between 400 and 1500 m, women were swimming faster than the men of 1968. The main graph shows, rather like that of skating, the extreme linearity in recent years of the time-distance plot over the range 400–1500 m, with a time-invariant intercept representing a store that cannot be fully used up in 100 or 200 m. The

Table 7.3 *Extrapolations of world records for women to the year 2000*

Distance (m)		Actual 1980	Extrapolated 2000
	60	7.2 s	6.87 s
	100	10.88	10.77
	200	21.71	21.35
	400	48.60	45.49
	800	1:53.5	1:44.42
	1500	3:52.47	3:42.13
mile	1609.35	4:21.7	4: 0.94
	3000	8:27.2	8: 2.27
	5000	15:08.8	13:52.84
	10 000	31:45.4	28:46.31
Marathon	42 195	2 h 27:33	2 h 14:36. 8

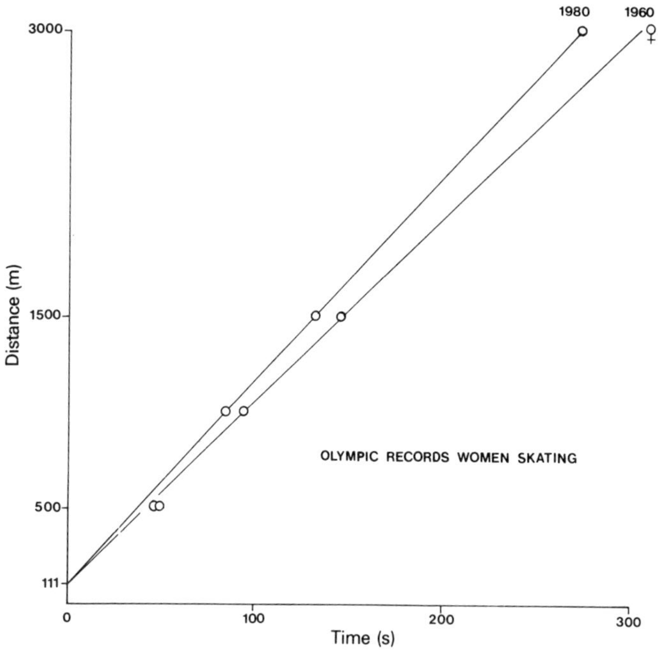

Fig. 7.7. Distance (m) plotted against time (s) from Olympic records for women skating, 1960–1980.

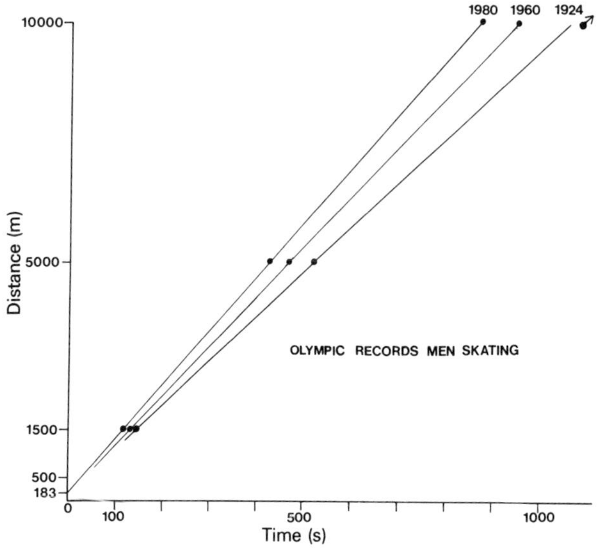

Fig. 7.8 Distance (m) plotted against time (s) from Olympic records for men skating, 1924–1980.

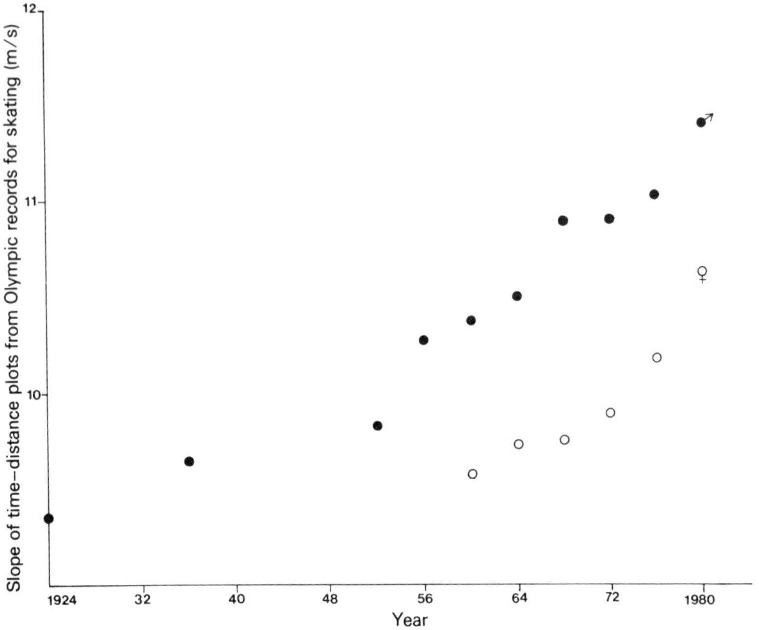

Fig. 7.9. Slopes of time–distance plots for Olympic skating record-holders 1924–1980, men ● and women ○.

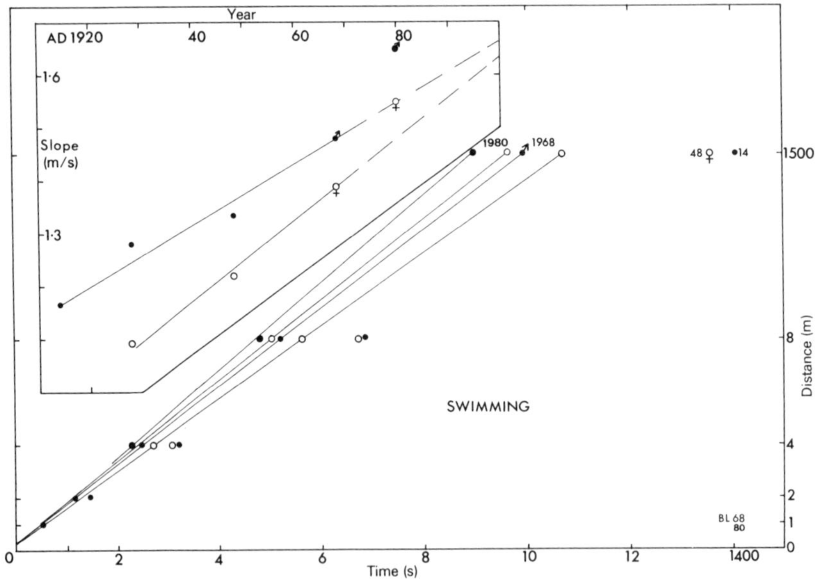

Fig. 7.10. World records: distance (m) plotted against time (s) for men ● and women ○ from 1914 to 1980. Inset. Slopes of lines for men and women plotted against calendar year.

slopes, plotted in the corner insert of Fig. 7.10, show an astounding increase for both men and women. These graphs were originally plotted in 1968 and have had the values for 1980 added. The dotted lines indicating development towards AD 2000 were drawn in 1968, and it will be seen that by 1980 women had moved on to the male line, and the men had leapt far above it. The trend to AD 2000 is unpredictable.

An interesting anomaly in swimming is that, compared with the trend in world records, the winning time for the men's 100 m at Mexico City in 1968 was relatively fast, in spite of the high altitude (2270 m above sea level) and the consequent shortage of oxygen. This causes hyperventilation at a given level of work and presumably greater buoyancy in a swimmer, to such an extent that in the shortest race, which is more independent of oxygen that the others, the lack of oxygen is outweighed by the buoyancy.

Acknowledgement

The author is very grateful to Dr Trevor Gethins of Oxford Polytechnic for his essential work on the recent evaluation of the parameters of eqn (7.11) and for most valuable discussions.

References

Anonymous (Leading article) (1968). Running towards Olympus. *Lancet* **2**, 816–17.

Cavagna, G. A. and Kaneko, M. (1977). Mechanical work and efficiency in level walking and running. *J. Physiol.* **268**, 468–81.

Hill, A. V. (1928). Air resistance to a runner. *Proc. R. Soc. Lond. B.* **102**, 380–5.

Lloyd, B. B. (1966). The energetics of running: an analysis of world records. *Advmt. Sci., Lond.* **22**, 515–30.

—— (1967). World running records as maximal performances: oxygen debt and other limiting factors. *Circulation Res.* **20**, 218–26.

—— (1967). Theoretical effects of altitude on the equation of motion of a runner. In *Exercise at altitude* (ed. R. Margaria) pp. 65–72. Excerpta Medica, Amsterdam.

—— (1969). The champion athlete – limiting factors in record-breaking. *Proc. R. Soc. Med.* **62**, 1164–6.

—— and Moran, P. T. (1966). Analogue computer simulation of the equation of motion of a runner. *J. Physiol.* **186**, 18–20P.

—— and Zacks, R. M. (1972). Theoretical optimization of time–velocity relationships in running short and middle distances. *Arch. Fisiol.* **69** Suppl., 494–501.

Pugh, L. G. C. E. (1971). The influence of wind resistance in running and walking and the mechanical efficiency of work against horizontal or vertical forces. *J. Physiol.* **213**, 255–76.

Zacks, R. M. (1971). Quantitative aspects of the motion of a runner, D. Phil. Thesis, University of Oxford.

8 Drugs and the athlete

H. THOMASON

Throughout history man has opposed his fellows, friend and foe alike, in various forms of physical competition in an attempt to prove who is the best amongst them. From earliest time the chroniclers of these events, be they of a friendly or deadly nature, have noted that some have sought to improve or sustain their physical performance by the use of various chemical aids, usually taken in the form of food or drink.

Lord Porritt (1969) said

> Hoping to increase performance by the help of some chemical aid or doping has been a phenomenon attached to man's physical competition for centuries. Dope, as originally defined, was a nice thick liquid used either as a food or a lubricant or both. This was its initial quite innocuous definition. It then came to have a sort of snide interpretation meaning some sort of stupefying drug, an intoxicant liquid with a narcotic effect, and this is what is now called negative doping or the giving of substances which will decrease the production of energy. Nowadays this applies essentially to animals. Finally, it came to mean the exact opposite, where doping implies the giving of a substance which *increases* function – that is, it increases the production of physical energy, which is the direct opposite of the initial definition. This is an interesting transition which has not yet really been properly explained.

An initial point has to be made that drugs are not wholly bad; to date nobody in medical or scientific circles has been able to distinguish clearly the difference between a medicine and a drug. The *Oxford English Dictionary* refers to a 'drug' initially as an original simple medicinal substance, organic or inorganic, used alone or as an ingredient, and defines a 'medical substance' as one having healing properties. Of the drugs that will be mentioned in this paper, the majority are, in fact, invaluable medicines if they are used properly, therefore the *intent* with which these substances are used leads to their being regarded as either a medicine or a drug. Anyone using them not to heal but to improve performance I would regard as taking drugs and thus doping themselves. This line of thinking led Hollyhock (1969) to state,

> Thus is it that probably, after all, the drug is not what really matters so much as the person who is induced, persuaded or encouraged to take it. There is, therefore, a religious or moral side to the issue which is surely an enormous factor. It is impossible to conjure up the circumstances in which there will be no drugs available – and so long as there are drugs available some people or other will resort to them, for better or for worse. How drugs are used is therefore a matter of education, and largely of moral education, and this applies not only to drugs in athletes but it applies to drugging in other circumstances as well.

Therefore, for present purposes, 'doping' will refer to the use of drugs taken purposely to improve performance, and the term athletes will be taken to mean any kind of sportsmen or women and not just track and field competitors. I shall attempt to demonstrate, using evidence reported in a variety of ways, from learned scientific papers to rumour and speculation amongst sportsmen, that doping has been and is a part of the athletic scene. Even the Ancient Olympics were not exempt, for some competitors were reputed to have taken various doping aids that they hoped would enable them to go further, faster, or higher. The ability to understand the properties of, and have access to, various drugs including stimulants, albeit in their natural form, has been available to man for at least 3000 years (Hollyhock 1969).

Instances throughout history are many, but those that spring most easily to mind are, for example, from Roman times – gladiators and chariot horses were treated with various dopes to improve performance and, therefore, provide a better spectacle for the customers. The knights in medieval jousts took stimulants, especially after injury, so that they could continue to fight.

One must, however, remember that these were peoples whose values were naturally different from our own. One sees recorded from earlier civilizations the use of drugs to secure purely sensual pleasure, or for necessity to enable one to complete one's social function and thus ensure protection from one's enemies. For example, the reconnaissance scouts of a South American Indian tribe were reputed to have gone out for periods of three to four days, taking with them only a small pouch and a supply of drugs to sustain them. This may have been a mixture of cocaine and caffeine. It is surprising that this use of drugs over a sustained period did not go hand-in-hand with any deterioration in mental or physical performance. In fact the reverse was expected of their use. Hollyhock (1969) attempts to answer this apparent anomaly thus:

> Indeed the whole point of taking the stuff was to improve the nerves and endurance, likewise these people did not appear to suffer dependence or tolerance. Now, insofar as they were using cocaine (and some of them certainly were), this is a little surprising: with marijuana it might not be so surprising but with cocaine it is. This peculiar phenomenon is perhaps that old problem of the soil and the seed. These people were using cocaine in a society which had that usage regulated by social custom very closely – used for purposes of war, used in religious ritual, and used in celebrations and festivals as well. But always within a socially-acceptable code and always in a regulated manner. In these circumstances they were able to take substantial doses and then be off the drug for long periods.

The question of dosage was very important and Hollyhock (1969) goes on to talk about:

> tribes who were, as a matter of fact, not unsophisticated about this, for example, the Baluba tribesman, the Bantus of the Congo, were acquainted with the varying effects

at different doses; at one end of the scale they smoked marijuana for themselves for enjoyment, much as people now smoke cigarettes (or at least some do); at the other end of the scale they submitted criminals or their enemies, any of those whom they wished to torture, to an atmosphere of dense marijuna smoke in order to produce unconsciousness in what must have been one of the most unpleasant ways possible. Perhaps this is the earliest use of poison gas.

Taking note of this use of drugs within a social context, and having a mind to dosage and effect, let us turn to more modern times and the first recorded instances of drug use in competitive sport. It must be remembered at this stage that those whose infamous deeds are reported must have been aware of the effect of these drugs and what, they hoped, would be the result of using them. Therefore, unless it can be proved otherwise, the intent in the use of these drugs must have been to make the recipient perform better physically. In the context of how I view sport, then these people were attempting to gain an unfair advantage and were 'cheating'.

The following is an incomplete record of instances when competitors engaged in sport have been suspected of having, or were actually found to have, taken drugs to improve performance.

In 1865 some competitors in the Amsterdam canal swimming races were suspected of taking some form of dope.

From 1870 onwards, six-day cyclists were reputed to use a series of miracle compounds in addition to nitroglycerine and sugar cubes dipped in ether. These races were conducted non-stop for six days and nights, and riders were expected not only to stay awake from Monday morning to Saturday evening but to race – for in the 1891 event, C. Miller covered 3368 km. These races were then banned and re-appeared at New York's Madison Square Garden in 1894 as two-man races: one rode whilst the other ate or slept at the trackside.

In 1914 the riders Grenda and Goullet recorded, in the 142 hours of racing, a distance of 4439 km, which I think still stands as a record.

Riders had mystic preparations in little black bottles! According to Novich (1964), French riders used a preparation known in the trade as 'Caffeine Houdes' – and horse blood serum. Belgian riders still used sugar cubes wetted with a few drops of ether, sucked while held between the teeth as they raced. Most six-day riders drank black coffee mixed with peppermint flavouring and caffeine capsules from a thermos, while others preferred tea mixed with brandy, the dosage of caffeine or brandy increasing as the six days progressed. In the mile and five-mile sprints, an integral part of the six-day racing programme, nitroglycerine capsules were taken to diminish the intensity and duration of dyspnoea (difficult breathing) found so frequently in cyclists after violent sprints. Caffeine capsules, coramine, and strychnine were also used. Cocaine and heroin were frequently given to riders by their trainers, cocaine being the most widely used stimulant for professional cyclists. Its effectiveness depended on the dosage and method of administration.

Prize-fighters of yester-year were given strychnine tablets, sips of diluted solution of aromatic spirits of ammonia, drinks of honey and brandy in combination, or drinks of brandy alone, before and during a fight. Some fighters had their head, face, and neck sponged with champagne to pep them up – some of this precious fluid probably found its way into the fighter's mouth. This might have had a stimulating effect purely on a psychological basis. However, strychnine, an established central nervous system stimulant, had to be given in near toxic doses to produce the desired 'hopping effect' in a fighter. This is *passé* now in boxing and other sports, but strychnine is still a good rat poison.

Some prize-fighters were massaged by their trainers with ointment containing cocaine and cocoa butter. This might have provided some surface anaesthesia from blows as well as some general stimulating effect. The final remedy to keep a fighter in the competition was the running of a lighted taper down the back.

Along with the notorious pedestrian races, these sporting competitors were all involved with money prizes and betting. However, the amateurs of the day were not without blemish. In the 1904 Olympics, Tom Hicks, the eventual winner of the Marathon, had almost certainly taken strychnine. Also, in the 1908 Marathon, Dorlando Pietri was suspected of taking strychnine.

So the story goes on. Part of the mystique of cycling, especially professional cycling on the continent where big prizes abounded, was not just the use of drugs, but which concoctions had the trainer or 'soigneur' obtained for you that would help you to beat your rival? What the professional cyclists did, the amateur, and hopefully future professional would also do. Cycling entered the post-war years with a reputation for uncontrolled drug taking as part and parcel of the sport. These sportsmen were using drugs given to them by their advisers, and many of them in later life said they could not have completed the strenuous time-table of competition without them. This use of such drugs as strychnine and heroin leads me to wonder how and who arrived at the correct dosage levels. Was it just hit-and-miss, with a few possible fatalities, or were servants of science and medicine also involved? We will probably never know!

The accusations of doping in sport, especially in cycling, continued until, in 1960 in the Rome Olympics, Knud Jensen of Denmark died on the opening day whilst competing in the team time-trial races. Traces of ronicol, a vasodilator, and amphetamine, a stimulant, were mentioned in the autopsy report. This was in the year after the French Physical Education Association had set up the first anti-doping commission. Unsubstantiated reports about drug use by competitors at these Olympics Games, and the previous ones in Melbourne and Helsinki, abounded and resulting from this, the furore eventually raised by Jensen's death, and pressure from the International Federation of Sports Medicine (FIMS), the International Olympics Committee (IOC) decided to take some action regarding this apparent drug problem. At this time also, some experts in Italy reported that between 14 and 46 per cent of all cyclists registered positive in dope tests of the day: 14 per cent in junior races and 46 per cent in professional races. These dope tests were far less sophisticated than those employed today.

In 1961, Professor Ottani, an Italian, said that 88 per cent of First Division Soccer Clubs in his country used drugs in games and training. The Tokyo Olympics in 1964 were said to be the scene of unprecedented drug taking by athletes in many of the sports contested.

FIMS persuaded the IOC to test competitors in the team time-trial, the event in which Jensen had died four years' previously. As yet there were no rules against doping in the Olympics. The doctors concerned with this first-ever testing at such a prestigious event were encouraged by the efficiency of the procedure and, though only a small variety of inoffensive drugs were found, pressurized the IOC to go further in the future.

The French Minister of Youth and Sport had been responsible for introducing an anti-doping law in 1963. Belgium made doping a national offence in 1965. The first doping tests at an athletic event in Britain were carried out during the whole of the 14-day Tour of Britain Cycle Race ('Milk Race') in 1965. All officials, 'soigneurs', and riders were aware of the procedure, and the eventual furore that arose when three Spaniards and one Englishman were found to have produced urine samples containing traces of amphetamine has left a permanent memory on my mind. I was the official of the Institute of Sports Medicine who conducted those first tests and the reception I received at the hands of some of the sporting press and some riders and officials led me to think that I was the guilty party.

The British Cycling Federation has always had my warmest praise and admiration for introducing dope testing to their most prestigious event, and, following one or two further disqualifications, have, it is to be hoped, rid that race of the iniquitous presence of drugs.

On the soccer field, the World Cup competition of 1966 also saw routine dope testing of a random sample of competitors throughout the finals. The results proved negative in all cases.

After 1966 it seemed that drug taking was being discouraged by the introduction of dope testing to an increasing number of sporting events by an increasing the number of governing bodies of sport.

Then in 1967 in the most prestigious cycling event of all, the Tour de France, Tommy Simpson, an ex-world professional road-racing champion and Britain's best-ever professional road-race cyclist, collapsed and died on the thirteenth day of the race whilst cycling on a very difficult mountain stage. Traces of amphetamine drugs were found in capsules on his person and recorded as being present in the very delayed autopsy report of his death. Although this event rocked the sport of professional cycling, it is sad to report that even today some cyclists are still caught by the drug-testing procedures. It was also suggested that some cyclists had discovered ways of bypassing the sampling stage, actual evidence of which was found. In addition, the use of drugs of such a kind and in such a form that the testing procedures could not detect them was also reported.

Introduction of anti-doping legislation and testing in the Olympics started in 1968 in Mexico City. So the story goes on, and in 1970 at the World Weight-lifting Championship in Columbus, Ohio, eight of the winners were disqualified for taking amphetamines, the only drug tested for. In the 1972 Olympics, Rick Demont, USA winner of the 1500 m free-style, was stripped of his Gold Medal when traces of a vasodilator drug were found in his urine. He was an asthmatic and claimed that the drug, which contained ephedrine, had been prescribed for his complaint.

Various medical bodies associated with sport had, from the late 1950s to the 1960s, spoken out against drug taking in sport and called for legislation that would allow them, on behalf of sports governing bodies, to stamp out this insidious practice. Some governing bodies had until then either refused to believe that doping took place in their sport or, even more difficult to believe, said that what competitors did, providing they kept within the rules of their sport, was their own responsibility.

At a European Symposium, doctors involved with sport listed the sports in their own countries where dope taking was apparent or strongly suspected. The list included cycling, soccer, horse-racing, horse-jumping, eventing (riders and mounts), car rally drivers, athletics, track and field, swimming, boxing, shooting, and tennis. The British Association of Sport and Medicine, FIMS, and the IOC Medical Commission set up in 1966, all spoke out against doping and set down legislation to counter it. Many then hoped that, with this legislation and the apparent signs that doping was on the decline (seen in the decrease in positive samples taken from athletes), the problem had been overcome.

In the editorial of a special issue of the *British Journal of Sports Medicine*, devoted to the proceedings of a symposium on 'Doping in sport'. J. G. P. Williams (1969), Secretary-General of FIMS, concluded his comments thus:

> We may all hope that in a sense this publication can now mark the end of an era when the whole question of doping and dope tests was somehow lurid and sensational, and the beginning of an era when these issues are regarded as nothing more than one of the many problems caused by the pressures of international competition, which are being tackled quietly, efficiently, systematically, and, it would seem, successfully. There is, of course, one other relevant issue still to be sorted out, and that is the use of anabolic steroids, but that is another story.

Thus we enter the next phase of drugs and the athlete. In the early 1960s reports on the use of anabolic steroids amongst athletes started to occur with increasing frequency. Doping legislation did not cover these synthetic compounds and testing procedures were not available. Pressure from doctors, scientists, and athletes alike eventually resulted in the necessary legislation, and Professor Brooks and his co-workers, with financial assistance from the Sports Council, developed techniques capable of detecting the use of these drugs (Sumner 1974; Brooks, Firth, and Sumner 1975) (see also Chapter 9). However, from 1960 to 1975 is a very long period in athletic terms.

The first use of these drugs to induce weight gain in athletes, rather than in under-nourished or anorexic patients, is attributed to the body-builders of California. Unconfirmed reports of their use by certain heavy-weight event athletes from the USA were circulating in 1960 and by the Olympics of 1964 many large competitors had become not only larger but very much more aggressive. Records in men's field events were broken with recurring frequency and after the 1966 Commonwealth Games in Jamaica, one of Britain's top, and certainly most senior field events competitors, Payne (1966) wrote:

> In terms of athletic morals it is better that we remain poor in the field events rather than that we achieve artificial results through doping. To my mind, the person who uses these anabolic steroids in athletics is as despicable as the cheat who knowingly uses a light discus in competition.

In a later paper (Payne 1975) he went on to say:

> This 1966 statement made me a lot of enemies at the time. From 1966 more and more British athletes began to 'experiment' with steroids. One of the typical explanations given by an athlete confessing that he had taken drugs is that he was 'just experimenting' – always against his better judgment.

Payne (1969) also stated that:

> In the 1968 Olympics I am sure that one of the factors involved in the magnificent performances was that the use of steroids had by then become widespread. It was rumoured that athletes in all events up to and including the 1500 metres in the American team were given steroids by their coaches. I have an impression, and it is only an impression, that up to until 1968, the world women athletes, and in particular the British women athletes, were relatively innocent, but from that time onwards that innocence began to die.

Witness the upsurge of female sporting success in, for example, East Germany, and the slower rise in West Germany. Discussions with defectors from East Germany, athletes, scientists, and doctors of sports medicine, by myself and others, lead me to conclude that the use of anabolic steroids, and other drugs, is part of the States' scientifically and medically-controlled sports training programme. Detection of anabolic steroids taken by female athletes from East European countries has taken place up to and including the last European Athletics Championships. Anyone who, like myself, witnessed on television the final of the women's long jump in the 1980 Moscow Olympics might, from the pictorial evidence presented, share my suggestion to the promotions manager of a certain company, which in that year withdrew its sponsorship from cricket because of lack of product identity with that sport, that he should think seriously about sponsoring women's athletics. The 'five o'clock shadow' on the face of the silver medallist would have done justice to any unshaven man.

It was hoped that the advent of the sophisticated techniques for detecting the presence of anabolic steroids in urine samples, would signal the end of the anabolic era. Far from it. Professor Beckett (1980), a member of the IOC Medical Commission, and others inform us that athletes are now switching to testosterone, the male sex hormone, after discontinuing the use of anabolic steroids before any games at which they know testing will occur. They conclude, correctly, that the testers will not be able to act because testosterone is endogenous to the body and, therefore, additional injected material cannot be detected. Professor Beckett admits that this is the current situation but is sure that before long this particular loophole will be plugged (see Chapter 9). At present, then, athletes are certainly taking drugs in an attempt to aid their performance. The legislation of the IOC and other governing bodies and the detection techniques seems usually to be a little behind what, it is supposed, some athletes are currently using. This has led Pickering (1979) to comment that some athletes may be taking more time finding out about the latest non-detectable drug than actually training.

Beckett and Cowan (1979) wrote:

> The function of dope control in sport is to constitute a deterrent, rather than to be punitive in its approach. Some people remark that there are few people caught in dope controls and therefore question the need for such control. For instance, they quote that of the 2079 urine samples collected in Munich only nine positive results were obtained and, of these nine, seven results led to disqualification. At Montreal there were three positive results in the conventional dope control and eight positive results in the anabolic steroid control.

There are many more examples of athletes taking anabolic steroids. In the West they seem to take the latest derivative without medical or scientific control. What would any doctor say if one of his colleagues distributed drugs without recourse to dosage or effect? This apparently uncontrolled taking of steroids and similar drugs is sure to lead to a more dangerous situation with regards to side-effects than if the use was properly controlled. What evidence there is in the West is scant; little scientific work has been carried out in the form of controlled experiments using these drugs with practising athletes. We are led to believe that this is not so in the Eastern bloc where controlled application, dosage, training, and even de-training and withdrawal, is practiced by the scientists and doctors attached to sports medicine. If this is so then their athletes may not be so much at risk. The situation is also constantly changing; thus Fulder (1980) writes:

> One drug which Soviet athletes undoubtedly used to increase their performance at the Olympics Games this year is a unique material which eludes classification or identification with any established categories of pharmaceutical substances. . . . it has not been included in the list of drugs which are banned for international sports events, nor is it in any Western pharmacopoeia.
>
> It is extracted from a plant of the same family as the ginseng root. Its properties include the ability to increase arousal and stamina without the side-effects that stimulants, such as amphetamines, caffeine or strychnine, have on the body.

The legislature laid down by the IOC regarding doping is hard enough pressed to keep pace with the latest in drugs. How will it handle this sort of development or any others that are bound to come from countries where scientists are encouraged to work in this area of science and human performance?

Reflect also on the comments in 1978 of the President of the European Athletic Association (Gold 1980):

> I have been reliably informed that in the recent Commonwealth Games in Edmonton, management officials of two large teams not only connived with, but actively assisted, some of their athletes to evade doping controls. Learning that there would be random testing on arrival in the village, they kept their athletes out of the village as long as possible and, in the case of one team, treated possible positives with diuretics and systematically flushed them with vast quantities of fluid.

If officials condone drug taking in attempts to improve performance, what hope is there for the individual athlete hoping to make the international team and then to do well against the competition? If the athlete is also backed by a powerful state system, then there may seem to be no place for an individual athlete who does not take drugs.

The International Amateur Athletic Federation (IAAF) first introduced an anti-doping rule as far back as 1928. More recently their anti-doping rules have, in keeping with the IOC Medical Commission, been strengthened by defining more closely what is meant by doping and incorporating a list of doping substances, anabolic steroids having been included since 1970.

In 1975 F. W. Holder, Honorary Secretary of IAAF, stated:

> Furthermore, the penalties for using dope have been increased. A guilty athlete is not only disqualified from the competition where the offence is detected, but also becomes ineligible to take part in competitions under IAAF rules. He is, therefore, effectively banned for life.
>
> Without doubt the main reason for introducing anti-doping rules in IAAF was to uphold the principle of fair play. The harsh discipline imposed on offenders may be partly due to the deceitful nature of the offence but has certainly been reinforced by the knowledge that doping can have lasting ill-effects on athletes and must therefore not be allowed to become prevalent.

These are sound words but, unfortunately, they have not been backed up with sound action. Ilona Slupianek of East Germany won the World Cup Women's Shot in Dusseldorf in 1977. Subsequently she was found to have taken anabolic steroids and was banned for 12 months. The ban finished two days before the European Championship in 1978 in Prague, where she won the Gold Medal. Some say that this 12-month ban had effectively given her time to train without any possible chance of detection.

Just prior to the Moscow Olympics, the President of the IAAF used his casting vote to allow four female competitors previously banned for taking steroids to compete in the Games. What price then the statement by his Honorary Secretary in 1975 'that the athlete is therefore effectively banned for life'?

These are some of the actions of the governing bodies of sport who are there, supposedly, to uphold all that is good within the sport. Surely drug taking cannot be so regarded. What chance have we to educate the young athletes of the future away from drug taking when officials, trainers, some doctors, and, of course, athletes are all involved in this pharmaceutical competition? Some say that the golden sands of California are second only to the golden triangle in Thailand.

You will hear today of the desirable and undesirable effects of steroids, the detection and monitoring of drug use in sport, and blood doping: is it management or manipulation? A young athlete at my own University is known as the number one non-anabolic steroid taker in his event in this country and he is only five in the rankings.

Which leads me to my final statements. Drug taking by athletes is not new, but the range of products taken has now reached ridiculous proportions. I was recently approached by a drug company to test the efficiency of a beta-blocker they produce by using our University athletes. The spokesman for the drug company said he was aware that the product was used by athletes and he wanted to know what effect it would have on performance. We declined to be involved.

It seems therefore that the pharmaceutical games are with us. The scientists and doctors in the West are criticized by many in sport for not detecting the latest drug being used. Unfortunately, I feel that the answer does not lie in this direction; the race between tester and athlete will not only be long and expensive in monetary terms but could eventually be so in lives.

We should rather take note of Payne's concluding comments after the 1968 Olympics (Payne 1969):

Perhaps we should emphasise the ethics of the situation, that drug taking is *cheating*, right from the start, instead of harping on the harmful side-effects. We should have cared about sport as a whole, rather than the damage a stupid athlete was inflicting on himself in his greed for glory – we should have pointed out and tried to educate people that the important thing in sport is to compete honourably, that to win at all costs is a contradiction of the meaning of sport.

In fact, Britain's number one pole vaulter in 1974 questioned whether top-class athletics could still be called sport, in the true sense of the word (Bull 1974): 'There are so many pressures now on international athletes that even in Britain the good loser is no longer accepted as a good sportsman.'

There is evidence to suggest that professionalism in sport seems to increase drug taking, e.g. professional cycling, American pro-football, and professional tennis. What chance track and field if it goes professional with agents and promoters, and schedules to meet not just weekly but sometimes daily?

Perhaps now is the time for us to step back and look anew. Britain was responsible for initiating and/or formalizing many of the modern sports played today. The idea of starting afresh and ensuring that our sportsmen play without the aid of drugs is not new; who knows but that more may follow, because if they do not then modern sport is heading along a road that I, for one, do not wish to follow.

References

Beckett, A. H. (1980). Dope detection at the Olympic Games. *Medisport* **2**, 168–72.

—— and Cowan, D. A. (1979). Misuse of drugs in sport. *Br. J. Sports Med.* **12**, 185–94.

Brooks, R. V., Firth, R. G., and Sumner, N. A. (1975). Detection of anabolic steroids by radio-immunoassay. *Br. J. Sports Med.* **9**, 89–92.

Bull, M. (1974). Philosophy of sport: *sic et non. Ath. Coach* **8**, 4.

Fulder, S. (1980). The drug that builds Russians. *New Scientist* **87**, 576–9.

Gold, A. (1980). (President of the European Athletic Association, 11th September 1978). In *Dope* (ed. L. Woodland). David and Charles, London.

Holder, F. W. (1975). Anabolic detection and enforcement. *Br. J. Sports Med.* **9**, 98–9.

Hollyhock, M. (1969). The application of drugs to modify human performance. *Br. J. Sports Med.* **4**, 119–27.

Novich, M. M. (1964). Use and misuse of drugs to improve athletic performance. *Proc. Int. Cong. Sports Sciences*, Tokyo, pp. 269–75.

Payne, A. H. (1966). Impressions of the discus throwing at the Jamaica Games. *Discobolus* **19**, 6.

—— (1969). Steroids. AAA Club Newsletter, 23 July 1969. Reprinted: *R. Can. Legion's Coach. Rev.* **7**, 1–14.

—— (1975). Anabolic steroids in athletics. *Br. J. Sports Med.* **9**, 83–8.

Pickering, R. (1979). Drugs in sport. *Sports Council Report* – Seminar for Governing Bodies of Sport, 13 December, pp. 10–16.

Porritt, A. (1969). Doping in Sport. *Br. J. Sports Med.* **4**, 105–8.

Sumner, N. A. (1974). Measurement of anabolic steroid by radioimmunoassay. *J. Steroid Biochem.* **5**, 307.

Williams, J. G. P. (1969). Special editorial for symposium proceedings on Doping in Sport. *Br. J. Sports Med.* **4**, 104.

9 Detection of steroid administration to athletes

R. V. BROOKS

Introduction

The use of synthetic anabolic steroids has been banned by most of the world's athletic and sporting organizations. Enforcement of this ban is by way of a two-stage testing procedure. First, urine samples from a relatively large number of athletes are subjected to a radioimmunoassay screening test. Any positive samples from this test are then examined by gas–liquid chromatography/mass-spectrometry to provide confirmation and to identify the particular anabolic steroid used. The complete test thus combines the high throughput and economy of radioimmunoassay with the virtual certainty of mass spectrometry.

The nature of anabolic steroids

Anabolic steroids are chemical modifications of the male hormone, testosterone. Testosterone has two, largely separate, types of action: by its androgenic activity it promotes the development of the male accessory reproductive glands and the secondary sexual characteristics such as the distribution of hair, voice changes, and certain behavioural effects, including an increased aggressiveness. However, there is also a second, more general action – an anabolic effect. This causes growth of the muscles. The anabolic steroids have structural changes to enhance the anabolic effect relative to the androgenic effect, although they all have some androgenic activity. Modifications which enhance this ratio of anabolic to androgenic effect (Fig. 9.1) are:

(1) The introduction of an additional double bond into the ring structure between C atoms numbers 1 and 2, as in methandienone (trade name Dianabol);
(2) attachment of a hydroxymethylene group at carbon 2, as in oxymetholone (trade names Anapolon or Adroyd);
(3) a pyrazole ring attached at carbons 2 and 3 as in stanozolol (trade names Winstrol or Stromba).
(4) the omission of the methyl group between the first two rings to give 19-nor steroids as in norethandrolone (trade name Nilevar) or ethylestrenol (trade names Maxibolin or Orabolin).

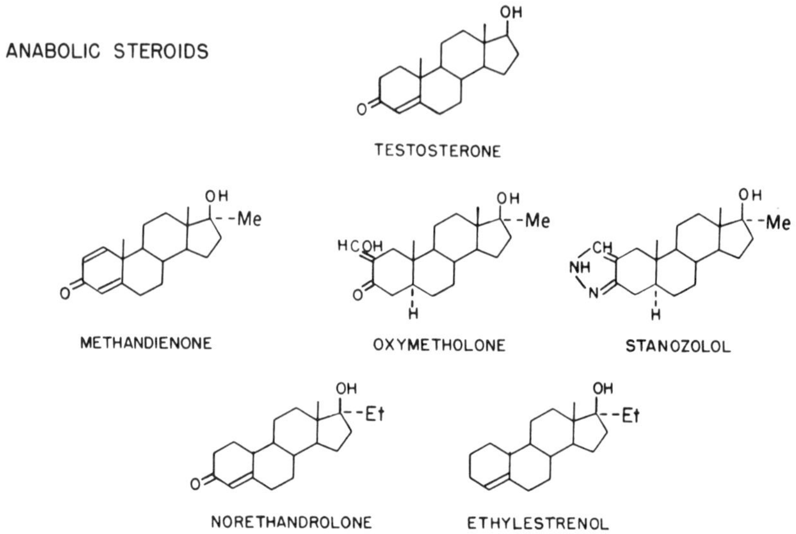

Fig. 9.1 Structural changes of anabolic steroids.

Orally active anabolic steroids have an additional modification in the presence of a methyl or an ethyl group attached at carbon 17. When anabolic steroids without such a group are taken by mouth, they are absorbed by the gut and taken to the liver in the hepatic portal blood where rapid inactivation takes place. The presence of the ethyl or methyl group at carbon 17 prevents the oxidation of the hydroxy group also attached to this carbon atom, and therefore prevents the inactivation of the steroid.

When we began to search for a screening technique to detect anabolic steroids, in the early 1970s, the orally active anabolic steroids with a 17α-alkyl group were the type being used by athletes: in particular methandienone, stanozolol, and norethandrolone. Eventually we turned to radioimmunoassay which, by this time, was being applied to smaller molecules such as steroids, having been in use for some years for large molecules such as the protein hormones.

Radioimmunoassay

The principle of radioimmunoassay is as follows. Unlike the natural steroid hormones the protein hormones vary in structure from species to species. When a protein hormone from one species is injected into a different species, antibodies may be produced. The antisera produced by this second species can be used as a reagent for measuring the hormone. Also needed for this assay system are a pure sample of the hormone to be measured (as a standard) and a sample of the hormone labelled with a radioactive isotope –

^{125}I- or ^{131}I-labelling of the tyrosine units in the protein is usually used. If a dilution of the antiserum is taken so that the amount of antibody is limited, and this is reacted with some of the radioactive hormone and a non-radioactive hormone standard, there will be competition between the labelled and unlabelled hormone. The hormone–antibody complex can be separated from the unreacted hormone by a variety of techniques, and the distribution of radioactivity between the two fractions can be measured. Clearly the more of the non-radioactive hormone present the smaller will be the proportion of bound radioactivity. If a graded series of standards is set up containing increasing amounts of unlabelled hormone with a fixed amount of radioactive hormone and antiserum, a standard curve can be drawn. As the amount of standard hormone increases so the amount of radioactivity bound, decreases. Unknown samples can then be assayed against this standard curve.

Unfortunately, steroid molecules are too small to be antigenic. However, if a steroid is firmly attached to a pure protein by covalent links and then injected into a foreign species (i.e. one foreign to the protein), antibodies will be produced. The surprising fact is that some of the antibodies produced are specific against the free steroid. We can, therefore, have a radioimmunoassay for the free steroid and use as the radioactive indicator either the ^{3}H-labelled steroid or a steroid–protein conjugate labelled with ^{125}I.

Although the preparation of antisera is still perhaps rather more art than science, one of the generalizations that has emerged is that the specificity of the antisera produced tends to be directed towards those parts of the molecule remote from the point of attachment of the steroid to the protein. As stated earlier, all the orally active anabolic steroids have either a methyl or an ethyl group attached to carbon atom number 17 at the right-hand end of the molecule, and in this they differ from all the natural steroid hormones. We thought that if we could direct the specificity to this right-hand end of the molecule by attaching it to the protein by the left-hand end, we might simplify the problem. We could then have one antiserum to detect all the 17α-methyl anabolics and another to detect all the 17α-ethyl anabolics (Fig. 9.2).

Screening test for orally active anabolic steroids

In the case of the 17α-ethyl steroids this approach was successful in that both the available 17α-ethyl anabolic steroids (norethandrolone and ethyl estrenol) cross reacted with the antiserum while the natural hormone, testosterone, did not.

The 17α-methyl antiserum cross reacted with all 12 available 17α-methyl anabolic steroids, although the percentage cross-reaction with some of them (notable stanozolol) was low. More seriously testosterone also cross-reacted

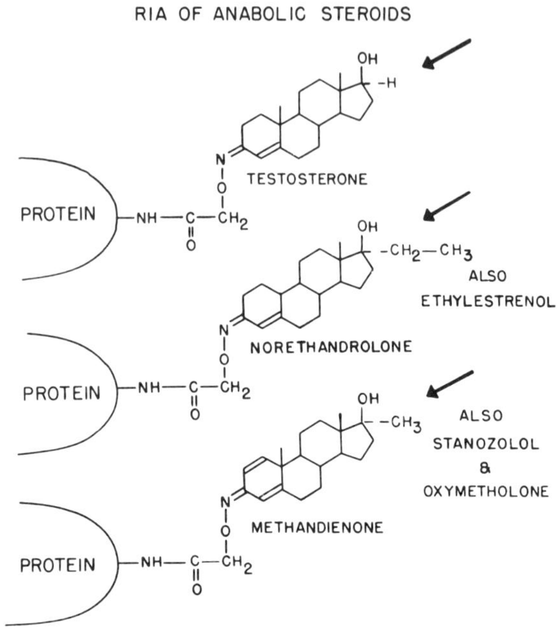

Fig. 9.2 Antigens for the preparation of group specific antisera to anabolic steroids.

to the extent of 4 per cent, an unacceptable degree of interference by the natural hormone. The cross-reaction was eliminated by acetylating the extracts before assay. Pyridine/acetic anhydride added to the dried extract converts all the testosterone to testosterone acetate which does not cross-react at all, but the 17β-hydroxyl group of the 17α-methyl steroids is sterically hindered, and so is not acetylated. The anabolic steroids are extracted from urine with an organic solvent (methylene chloride) without prior hydrolysis. Although hydrolysis would split the conjugates and release much larger quantities of anabolic steroid metabolites, some of which might react with the antiserum, this procedure would take time. Since the concentration of unconjugated testosterone is negligible in fresh urine specimens, the acetylation stage may be omitted and the assay of a batch of about 50 samples may then be completed in seven hours. The poor cross-reaction that the original antiserum (RN2) had for stanozolol could be improved somewhat by using charcoal adsorption to separate bound and free antigen instead of the original coated tube method (Table 9.1). A much bigger increase in the cross-reaction of this steroid was effected by using an antiserum raised in another rabbit to the same antigen (RN11). This gives a cross-reaction of 70 per cent with charcoal separation but the cross-reaction of testosterone has risen to 31 per cent. Fortunately the acetate still does not interfere.

Table 9.1 *Variation of specificity of antisera (17***a**-methyl testosterone-3-carboxymethyloxime-HSA-antisera) according to method of separation and batch of antiserum

	% Cross reaction at 50% displacement RN2		RN11	
	Charcoal	Coated tube	Charcoal	Coated tube
Methandienone	100	100	100	100
Testosterone	7.5	3.7	31	23
Testosterone Ac.	0	0	0	0
Stanozolol	7.1	3.2	70	50
Oxymesterone	67	46	105	62
Bolasterone	—	61	180	100
Nilevar	0	0	12	—

Anabolic steroids given by intramuscular (IM) injection

When the tests for the orally active anabolic steroids were brought into use in 1974 it seemed likely that athletes might turn to steroids such as Durabolin and Decadurabolin, which are effective only if given by intra-muscular injections. These are both esters of 19-nortestosterone, the function of the ester grouping being to delay absorption of the steroid from the site of injection and therefore reduce the frequency with which injections must be made. Since the 19-nortestosterone is not absorbed until the ester grouping is removed, it is only necessary to have an antiserum capable of recognizing 19-nortestosterone itself. 19-Nortestosterone differs from testosterone only in the absence of a methyl group between the A and B rings, i.e. at the left-hand side of the molecule.

It appeared therefore, that conjugation to the protein through the D-ring rather than the A-ring might give the best hope of the required specificity. The hemisuccinate of 19-nortestosterone was prepared and conjugated with human serum albumin. Immunization of rabbits with this antigen gave an antiserum which did not cross-react at all with testosterone. This was fortunate because, in this case, acetylation could not have been used to overcome the problem. This antiserum can also be used to detect administration of the two 17α-ethyl steroids (norethandrolone and ethyl oestrenol) so that only two antisera are needed for the complete radioimmunoassay screen.

As in the radioimmunoassay for orally active anabolic steroids, steroid ^{125}I-histamine labels were used. Due to their relatively short half life (60 days) these labels must be prepared at intervals of two to three months; nevertheless they have considerable advantages because of the simplicity and speed of counting. Also, some of the laboratories using our kits for carrying out tests have γ- but not β-counting facilities.

This test for Durabolin and Decadurabolin was used for the first time at the Olympic Games in Montreal in 1976. Surprisingly no positive results were found in this test, although there were eight positives for orally active anabolic steroids. At first we thought that we had misjudged the situation in supposing that athletes would turn to injected steroids. However, the following year, in the European Athletics cup, there were five positive results in the intramuscular test and only two for oral steroids. So much, then, for the journalists oft repeated claim that the cheats will always be several steps ahead of any measures intended to control them.

The screening test is very sensitive. The antiserum for the intramuscular steroids can pick up as little as 1 pg (i.e. 10^{-12} g) per tube. It has been claimed that positive urine tests have been obtained some months after the last dose of anabolic steroid was administered.

Confirmation by gas–liquid chromatography/mass spectrometry

The certainty of the testing procedure and the ability to identify the particular anabolic steroid which has been taken, depends on this last stage of the test. It is at present less sensitive than the screening test, requiring *more* urine sample and hydrolysis of the steroid metabolites. After some preliminary purification, the extract is fractionated on a gas chromatogram which resolves the complex mixture into its separate components. The identity of any one of these components can then be examined in the mass spectrometer, which splits the component into fragments which are focused according to their ratio of mass to charge. Thus a virtual 'fingerprint', characteristic of the component, is obtained.

This confirmation by mass spectrometry is more important in the test for injected steroids than it is for those given by mouth, because women taking certain contraceptive steroids may give a false positive in this screening test. We are at present trying to overcome this defect by preparing an antiserum to the major matabolite of 19-nortestosterone which is excreted in amounts several hundred times greater than those of the unchanged steroid.

The future of anabolic steroids abuse in athletics

Several pieces of evidence suggest that the benefits male athletes claim to get from anabolic steroids arise primarily from their androgenic rather than their anabolic action. If that is so, then it would surely be more sensible to take testosterone itself rather than one of the chemical modifications which tend to have more undesirable side effects. Since oral testosterone is about 98 per cent inactivated before reaching the general circulation, intramuscular injection of esters would appear to be the most likely method of administration.

Detection of the administration of the natural male hormone presents an entirely novel problem in the control of drugs in sport. Is is possible to set a limit for the rate of excretion of testosterone in urine beyond which administration of testosterone may be considered to have taken place? It would clearly be necessary to establish normal values for athletes and to examine the possibility of an effect of violent exercise on the excretion of testosterone. Concentrations of the hormone in blood would certainly provide a more valid basis for comparison than its excretion in the urine. However, athletes are, in general, unwilling to provide blood samples. Since accurately timed collections of urine are also out of the question here, some method must be found to allow for the wide variations which may occur in the degree of dilution of the urine.

The method which we have proposed and are in the process of testing utilizes the body's own control system as an indicator (Fig. 9.3). It depends on the fact that administration of testosterone in doses equal to or greater than the rates of endogenous secretion causes suppression of the pituitary secretion of luteinizing hormone. The ratio of the concentration of testosterone to that of luteinizing hormone would therefore appear to be a more sensitive index of administration of testosterone than would the concentration of either of them. If it were possible to measure this ratio in urine it might provide an ideal test since the ratio would be independent of the degree of urinary concentration.

We have tested this possibility in a group of ten volunteer medical stu-

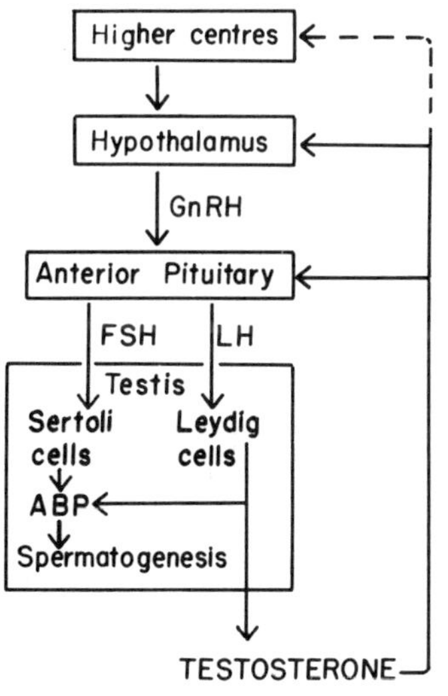

Fig. 9.3 Negative feed-back control of testosterone secretion: luteinizing hormone (LH) stimulates testosterone secretion, testosterone inhibits LH secretion.

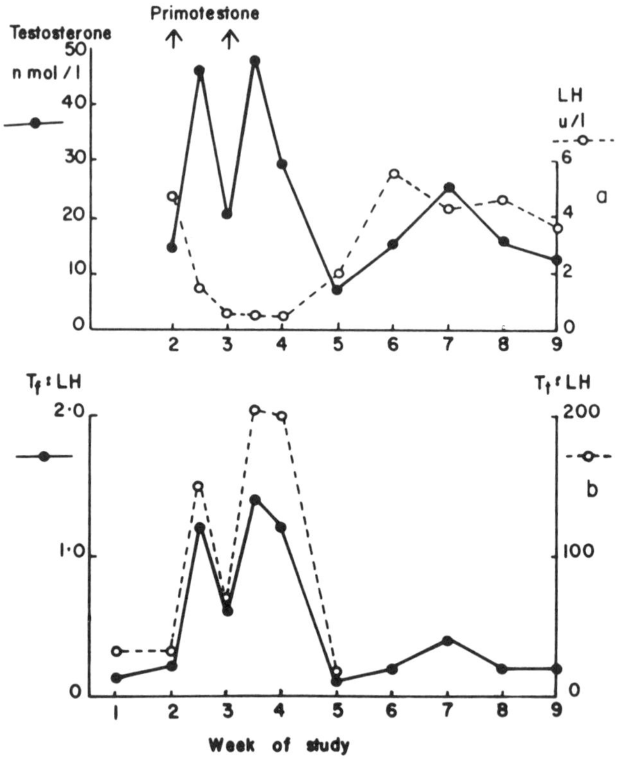

Fig. 9.4. Effect of injections of testosterone esters (250 mg) on the plasma levels of luteinizing hormone and testosterone in one subject. Injections were administered on completion of the urine and blood collections on weeks 2 and 3. Upper chart shows the plasma concentrations of testosterone ——●—— and luteinizing hormone (LH) — — O — —. Lower chart shows the ratios of free testosterone to luteinizing hormone (T_f : LH) ——●—— and total testosterone to luteinizing hormone (T_t : LH) — — O — — in the urine.

dents given 250 mg of testosterone esters on two occasions, either 1 week or 2 weeks apart. Typically (Fig. 9.4) the concentration of testosterone in the blood three days after the injection had doubled, but at seven days was only a little above the pre-injection level, while after 14 days it was less than half this concentration. This means that to secure any advantage, injections must be given at intervals of one week or less. Not only is the ratio of testosterone to luteinizing hormone altered proportionately more than the testosterone concentration, but because the luteinizing hormone remains depressed, the ratio gives a greater degree of retrospectivity. This short-term trial indicated that the blood hormone level is a more sensitive test than the level in the urine. However, with a longer course of injections, which would appear to be necessary to obtain any competitive advantage, the urine ratio should form an effective screening test. Possible means of confirmation include the ratio of testosterone to follicle-stimulating hormone in the urine and the ratio of ^{12}C to ^{13}C in the testosterone excreted in the urine.

10 What are the effects of anabolic steroids?

G. R. HERVEY

J. B. S. Haldane once commented that, somewhere in the mists of pre-history, the male gonads must have been the first targets of biotechnology. The functions of these organs have been progressively clarified by modern scientific study, with much benefit to medicine and agriculture. It is now appreciated that all the visible distinguishing features of the sexes are brought about by the actions of chemical messengers, the hormones, secreted by the respective gonads. These hormones have been chemically identified: together with the hormones of the adrenal glands and a large range of synthetic compounds they belong to the chemical family known as steroids (Fig. 10.1).

In what we tend to regard as 'normal' animals – since they include ourselves – males are larger and more muscular than females. There are, indeed species such as the hamster and chinchilla, in which the opposite is true; their hormones are much the same as man's. Disregarding them, however, it seems at first sight a reasonable assumption that the greater body size and muscularity of males are, like other male characteristics, produced

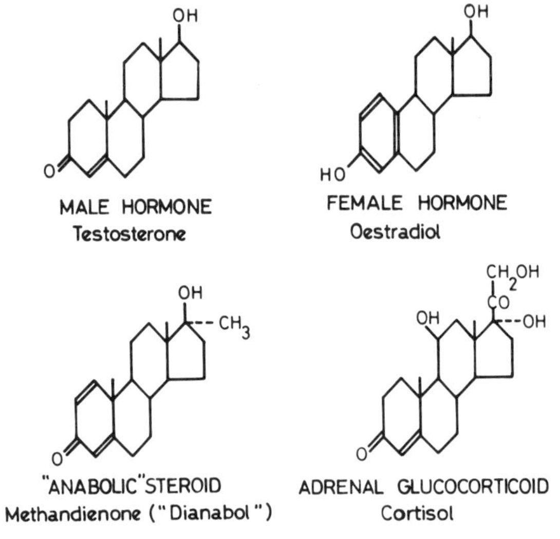

Fig. 10.1. Chemical formulae of steroids. These are conventionally drawn. The molecules are really egg-shaped.

by the action of the male hormone, testosterone. Testosterone must, therefore, have a muscle building, or 'anabolic' action. This conclusion was reached nearly fifty years ago (Kochakian and Murlin 1935). It has provided the basis for some use of 'anabolic steroids' in medicine and rather more in agriculture, and for their use, or abuse, in sport.

It is unfortunately true that, although experiments should be designed to have the best chance of disproving the experimenter's starting hypothesis, in practice he tends to find what he is looking for. The experiments of a generation ago with rats – the species in which the endocrine system has been most studied – appeared to confirm that testosterone had the expected anabolic action. Figure 10.2 illustrates a fair example. By modern standards this experiment is open to criticism. We are not shown how the rats' weights were changing before treatment; there are no untreated or solvent-treated control groups; most importantly, the latter part of the 'observed' weight graph shows a fall, which suggests that the rats might have finally shown a weight loss if treatment had not been stopped. (The author refers to 'wearing off' of the effect of the hormone, but does not attempt to reconcile this with the proposition that it reproduces a normal male characteristic. The dotted line may have been thought to illustrate anabolism better, but it could also be held to illustrate the hazards of using 'corrected' rather than real physiological data, and the difficulties of measuring nitrogen balances.)

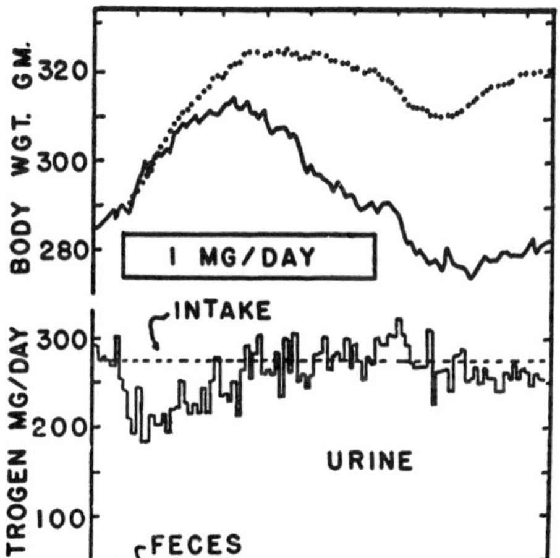

Fig. 10.2 Experiment reported by Kochakian (1950). The caption read: 'Effect of prolonged injections of testosterone propionate on body weight and nitrogen excretion of castrated rats (Wistar). The observed body weights are graphed as a solid line. Body weight calculated from the nitrogen retained is shown by the dotted line'.

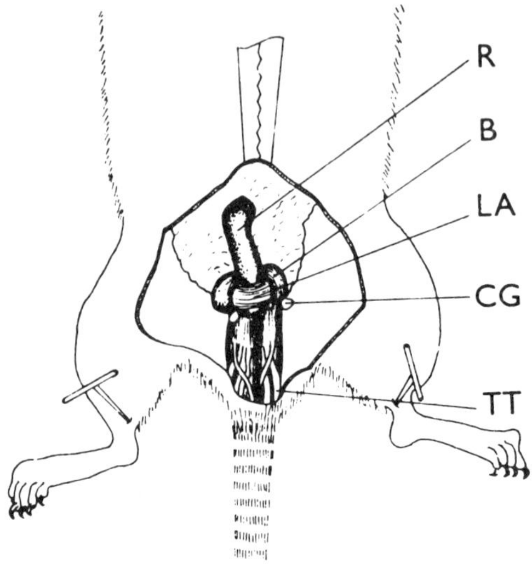

Fig. 10.3. The rat 'levator ani' (Rassaert, Wolff, and McDougal 1968). R, rectum; B, bulbocavernosus; LA, levator ani; CG, Cowper's gland; TT, tail tendons.

The apparent demonstration of the anabolic action of testosterone led to much activity by the pharmaceutical industry. This was directed towards synthesizing analogues of testosterone in which, as had been possible in other instances, actions of the natural hormone were separated; in this case the hope was to separate the supposed anabolic action from the androgenic actions (i.e. the familiar effects upon reproductive structures). The 'anabolic' steroids were the outcome.

Screening of large numbers of potential drugs called for a simple, rapid test. It seemed reasonable to use the weight of a single excised muscle as a measure of an effect upon muscles in general. With hindsight, it seems surprising that the difficulty of finding a suitably responsive muscle did not prompt the investigators and subsequent users of the test to look more critically at the one supposedly found; particularly since subsequent studies of numerous individual muscles in the rat and guinea pig showed little effect of testosterone treatment on any of them (Kochakian and Tillotson 1957; Kochakian, Tillotson, and Endahl 1956). The responsive muscle was the rat's 'levator ani' (Fig. 10.3), and it became the basis of the standard test for 'anabolic' activity (Eisenberg and Gordan 1950). It is not, in fact, homologous with the human muscle of the same name, an important skeletal muscle in the pelvic floor, but is part of the male reproductive tract, and also known as the dorsal bulbocavernosus (Hayes 1965). Nevertheless, the change in weight of this muscle was widely used to measure 'anabolic' activity and supposedly to distinguish it from androgenic activity, which was measured by the weight of the seminal vesicles. Books were written on the relationship

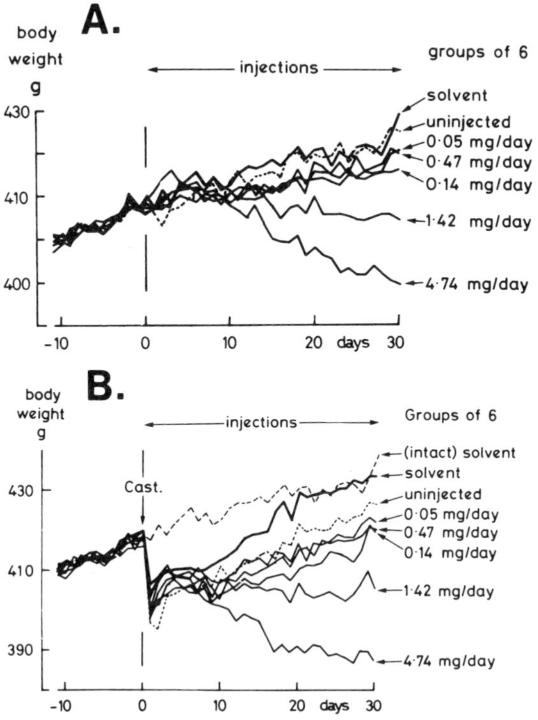

Fig. 10.4. Body weight graphs of (A) intact and (B) castrated male rats, 6 months old, of the inbred WAG/C × PVG/C strain, given testosterone daily in the doses shown for 30 days. Doses were subcutaneous, in 0.1 ml arachis oil. 'Solvent' group received 0.1 ml oil only. 'Uninjected' group received no injections.

of chemical structure to 'anabolic:androgenic ratios' so measured (Krüskemper 1968; Vida 1969). The compounds selected were confidently advertised.

Our interest in the 'anabolic steroids' arose from a longstanding interest in the effects of other steroids on the weight and composition of the body: for example, the mechanism by which steroids from the ovaries cause energy to be stored as fat in early pregnancy (Hervey 1969; Hervey and Hervey 1967, 1981). The 'anabolic' effect and the sex difference in body size were clearly interesting in themselves; we also hoped that better understanding of the effects of synthetic anabolic steroids would contribute to an informed approach to the difficult problems created by their use by athletes.

My colleague Ian Hutchinson was particularly concerned in studies of the effects of testosterone, and of related natural and synthetic steroids, on body weight and composition in the rat (Hervey and Hutchinson 1972; Hutchinson 1978). The changes in weight and composition were measured by accurate methods that we had developed for studies of female

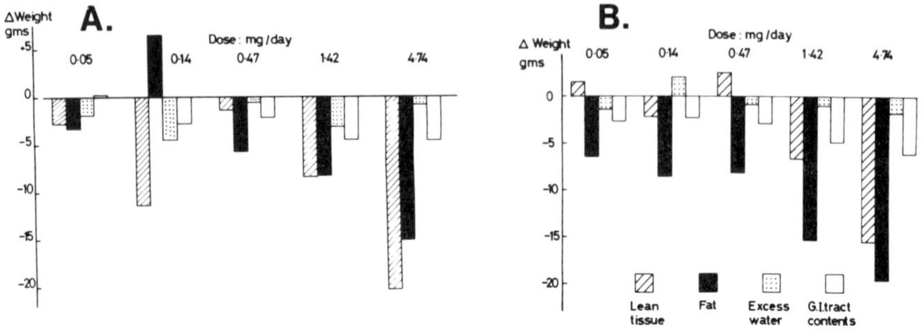

Fig. 10.5. Changes in body composition in the experiment shown in Fig. 10.4. Changes over the treatment period were measured from differences between treated and control groups found by carcass analysis at the end of the experiment, with adjustments applied for the small differences between the starting weights of the groups. The analysis divided the terminal live weight into four components: lean tissue comprises the non-fat solids, mainly protein and minerals, together with water in the proportion found in the lean bodies in the control group; fat is extractable lipid; excess water is any change in water additional to that included in 'lean tissue'; and the contents of the gastrointestinal tract. Gain or loss of each constituent is shown by the length of a bar drawn up or down from the zero line.

hormones. Figures 10.4(A) and 10.4(B) show the changes in body weight in male rats, with and without their gonads, when given testosterone in a range of doses.

If anabolic action exists, castrated male rats should provide the most sensitive test for it. Castration itself, however, did not appreciably alter body weight; nor did treatment of intact or castrated rats with testosterone in doses up to the physiological replacement dose, which is about 1 mg/day given in this way. Higher doses led to loss of weight. Analysis of the bodies showed no changes in composition up to the physiological dose; lean tissue and fat were lost at higher doses (Fig. 10.5).

Ovariectomized female rats showed similar changes to males. In intact female rats there was a suggestion that testosterone produced an increase in lean tissue, at the expense of fat and with no overall change in weight. This can hardly be regarded as evidence for a normal action of testosterone exerted in the male; a parallel for it will be mentioned later some biologically related compounds investigated caused weight changes with a similar pattern, but less pronounced. A typical synthetic 'anabolic steroid' also had effects similar to those of testosterone (Fig. 10.6).

Hutchinson also showed that the rat 'levator ani' muscle underwent the same pattern of weight changes in response to castration and to graded doses of testosterone as did other reproductive structures, such as the seminal vesicles. On the other hand, individual skeletal muscles showed the same pattern as the body as a whole (Fig. 10.7).

The question then arose: if testosterone does not change body size, how do male rats become larger than females? Another colleague, John Harvey,

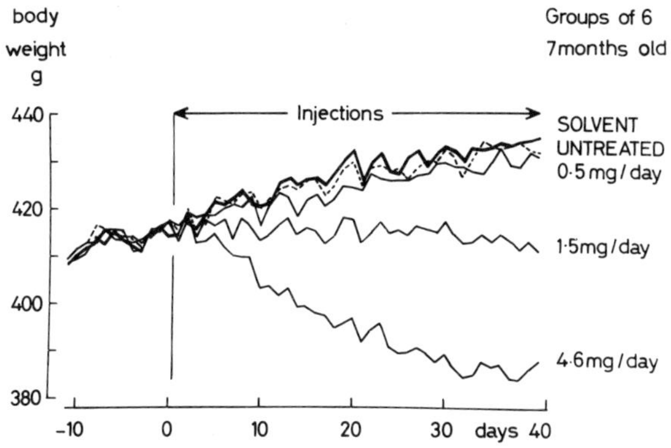

Fig. 10.6. Body weights of male rats given the synthetic anabolic steroid methandienone (Dianabol) daily in the doses shown. Methods as for testosterone experiment.

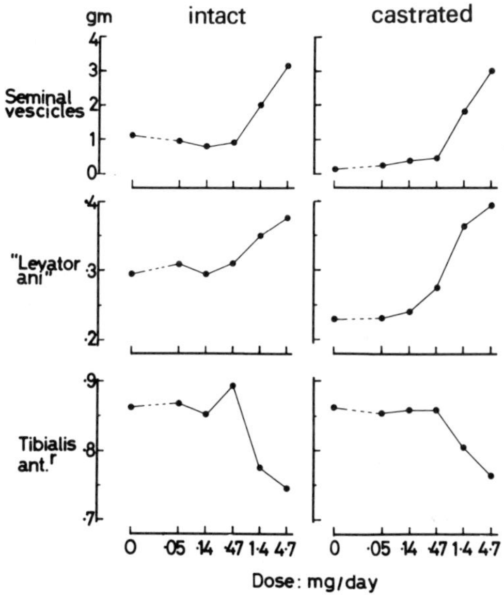

Fig. 10.7. Organ weights in male rats, intact and castrated, given testosterone in a range of doses for 30 days. Means of six 6-month old rats. Note the difference between organ weights in intact and castrated rats at zero dose; the effects in each case of doses of testosterone up to 0.47 mg/day; and the effects of higher doses.

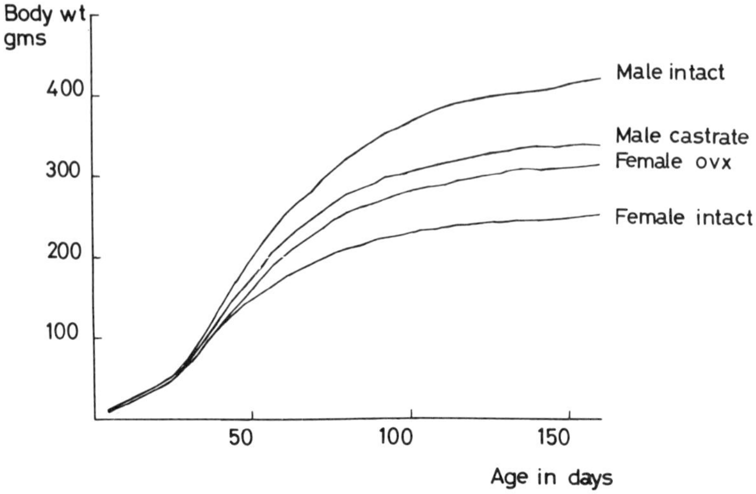

Fig. 10.8. Body weight graphs of male and female rats, intact and gonadectomized on the day of birth. Male hormone increases body weight, female hormone reduces it, and the sum of the effects accounts for the adult sex difference in weight. Note, however, that removing the gonads later in life shows that male hormone exerts its effects, on subsequent growth, irreversibly and only during the short period after birth; the action of female hormone is exerted continuously during adult life and is lost if the hormone is withdrawn.

investigated this (Harvey, Hervey, and Hutchinson 1972; Harvey 1976). It was already known that the rat's brain is sensitive to testosterone for a short time after birth. In males, testosterone is secreted briefly at this time; its action then causes the patterns of control of gonadal hormone secretion and of sexual behaviour, which are developed later, to be those characteristic of the male. By removing the gonads soon after birth, Harvey was able to show that testosterone similarly switches the pattern of body growth, in advance and irreversibly, to the male pattern. Interestingly, the pattern for future growth is sensitive to the level of nutrition at the same critical time. In rats the ovaries also contribute to the sex difference in weight; the action of their hormones is to reduce body weight; but this is exerted at the time the hormones circulate and is reversible. The sum of the two effects approximately accounts for the sex difference in body size in adult rats (Fig. 10.8).

Our experiments with rats thus totally failed to confirm all the premises on which the use of 'anabolic' steroids by humans had been based. Since it was known that many athletes took steroids and evidently were convinced of the anabolic action, it seemed of interest and justifiable to attempt to measure the effects in man. This was done in two experiments by a strong interdisciplinary team, in which Alec Knibbs and Lewis Burkinshaw made major contributions (Hervey 1975; Hervey, Hutchinson, Knibbs, Burkinshaw,

Jones, Norgan, and Levell 1976; Hervey, Knibbs, Burkinshaw, Morgan, Jones, Chettle, and Vartsky 1981).

In each experiment, after the purpose and procedures of the experiment had been explained, about a dozen male athletes volunteered to take methandienone (methandrostenolone; Dianabol) in a dose of 100 mg/day for six weeks. This is typical of the doses taken by athletes and is by no means the maximum. Both experiments were double-blind and crossed-over: that is, there were two six-week periods of treatment, separated by six weeks; a subject received the drug during one period and dummy tablets ('placebo') during the other; the order in which the two treatments were given varied among the subjects and was unknown to them or to the observers.

During each treatment period the subjects pursued a course of weight training. In the first experiment the subjects had not trained previously at this activity. In the second experiment the subjects were competitive weight-lifters, and the treatments were superimposed on their normal continuous training; they were also older than the subjects of the first experiment. A few subjects had to be withdrawn from the experiments, usually for failure to comply with the programme, but in one instance because of a rise in one of the blood enzyme concentrations used to monitor liver function. This was the only side-effect attributable to the drug.

The experiments were designed primarily to measure changes in body composition. There are various methods for doing this in living humans. These are inevitably less accurate than analysis of animal carcasses, but it is possible to use several methods and collate the results. In both experiments we measured: body weight; skinfold thickness, as a measure of body fat content; body density, which gives the proportion of lean tissue and fat; body potassium content, which measures cellular tissue; the circumference of limbs; and the thicknesses of limb muscles and of subcutaneous fat by X-rays. In the second experiment, through the co-operation of Professor Fremlin's Department of Physics at Birmingham, we were able to add measurements of body nitrogen, which reflects the body's protein content. All the methods other than the simple measurements involve assumptions that may not be valid if the composition of the body becomes abnormal.

Two measures of athletic performance were also recorded: the maximum load achieved in each of three weight-lifting exercises, which followed a standard increasing pattern; and the static strength of each of three groups of muscles, in the leg, arm, and hand. In the first experiment maximum oxygen consumption, which measures the capacity for work, was also measured. The subjects' medical condition was checked regularly.

The body composition studies, shown in Table 10.1, gave consistent results in the two experiments. Unlike the rats the subjects did gain weight when they took the drug, to the extent of 2–3 kg over the six weeks. Body density, body potassium, and in experiment 2 body nitrogen, the indicators

Table 10.1 *Changes in body composition and dimensions in experiments on man*

	Exp.	Initial value	Change on placebo	Change on drugs	Significance†
Body weight (kg)	1	77.3	−0.2	+ 3.3	**
	2	87.7	−1.3	+ 2.3	**
Body nitrogen (kg)	2	2.06	+0.04	+ 0.26	*
Body potassium (g)	1	180	−3	+16	**
	2	190	−2	+17	***
Lean body by density (kg)	1	68.4	−0.4	+ 2.4	**
	2	70.5	0	+ 3.1	***
Thigh circumference	1	568	−1	+13	*
(mm)	2	602	−6	+11	**
Arm circumference	1	308	0	+13	*
(mm)	2	354	−2	+11	*
Muscle widths by X-ray (3 muscles)	1	302	+4	+15	*
(2 muscles)	2	182	−3	+ 8	**
Fat by density	1	8.9	+0.2	+ 0.9	NS
(kg)‡	2	17.2	−1.2	− 0.8	NS

† From paired *t* test, applied to the differences between the changes on the placebo and on the drug. *, **, ***, significant at 5, 1, and 0.1 per cent levels respectively. NS = not significant.
‡ Fat by skinfolds and X-rays gave similar results to fat by density.

of lean tissue, all increased. Limb circumferences and X-rays showed increases in the size of muscles. Body fat, measured by skinfolds, density and X-rays, did not change significantly. Thus at first sight the experiments appeared to confirm the conventional view that anabolic steroids cause increased muscularity; surprising as this might seem to us in the light of our failure to confirm the animal evidence, which had provided the original basis for the use of the compounds.

Table 10.2 shows the changes in the measures of performance in the first experiment. Performance at weight-lifting and the strength of the leg muscles increased greatly over the experimental periods; but to the same extent whether drug or dummy had been taken. The improvement presumably reflected the effect of the new form of training. There was no effect upon maximum oxygen uptake.

Table 10.3 shows the changes in the second experiment. This time performance and strength increased over the period of treatment with the drug, but not when the dummy was given. The fact that the training programme continued throughout may have produced a more sensitive test. There is, however, a possibility that in those subjects who took the drug before the placebo, its effect might not have completely worn off by the start of the placebo period; this would produce an apparent negative change over the placebo period and so exaggerate the difference between treatments. In

Table 10.2 *Changes in performance in experiment 1*

Exercise	Initial value	Change on placebo	Change on drug	Significance†
Weight training (kg)				
Leg press	126	+60	+60	NS
Arm press	45	+15	+15	NS
Muscle strength (kg)				
Legs	394	+40	+42	NS
Hand	49	0	+ 1	NS
Work capacity				
$\dot{V}O_{2max}$ (1/min)	4.1	+ 0.1	+ 0.1	NS

† NS = not significant.

both experiments there was no change in the strength of the grip, which uses muscles not exercised by the training.

The evidence in the literature on the effects of anabolic steroids on athletic performance is equivocal. Howard Payne (1975) devised one of the best tests. He plotted the annual averages of the ten best world and UK performances in various sports against the year. Figure 10.9 reproduces four of these graphs. All show the progressive improvement in performance which characterizes so many human activities. The period covered spans the early 1960s, when the taking of steroids became prevalent; if steroids have a significant effect on performance, this should show as a change in the level or slope of the graphs. The contestants in the 10 000 m race (Fig. 10.9(A)) are unlikely to take steroids and no such change is evident. The graph for pole vaulting (Fig. 10.9(B)) does show an upturn in the early 1960s; this reflects the introduction of the fibreglass pole, and verifies the effectiveness of Payne's method. The graphs for discus throwing and shot putting, sports

Table 10.3 *Changes in performance in experiment 2*

Exercise	Initial value	Change on placebo	Change on drug	Significance†
Weight training (kg)				
Leg lift	138	+ 2	+16	**
Arm lift	114	+ 4	+17	*
Muscle strength (kg)				
Legs	419	−17	+68	*
Arms	92	+ 5	+13	NS
Hand	55	− 2	+ 3	NS

† From paired *t* test, applied to the differences between the changes on the placebo and on the drug. *, **, *** significant at 5, 1, and 0.1 per cent levels respectively. NS = not significant.

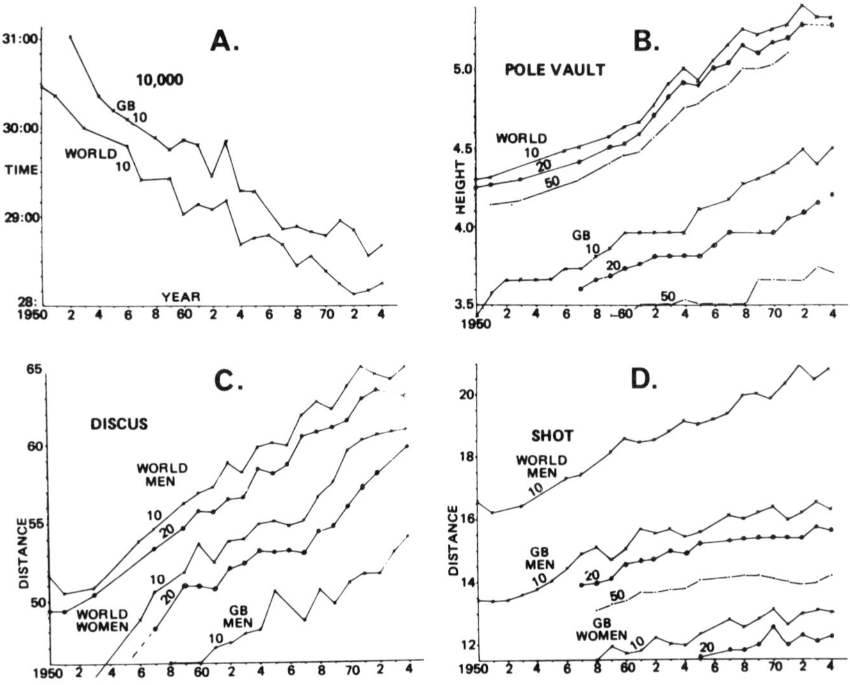

Fig. 10.9. Graphs drawn by Howard Payne (1975) showing attainment in various events, as means of the ten best world and British performances, plotted against the year. (A) 10 000 m race; (B) pole vault; (C) discus throwing; (D) shot putting.

notorious for the use of steroids, provide the test cases. It is left to the reader's eye to judge whether an effect is visible. Personally I am not convinced that it is.

Table 10.4 examines the implications of the gains of potassium and nitrogen produced by the drug. This has been done by listing the gains of weight with which these gains would be expected to be associated, on different assumptions as to the nature of the substance gained. It seems clear that the increased size of the muscles was not brought about by gain of normal muscle tissue. In both experiments the amount of potassium gained was almost twice the amount that would be expected if the gain had been normal muscle. The relationship between body potassium content and density was significantly shifted (Hervey *et al.* 1976), also indicating a change in the overall composition of the lean body. Taken by itself, the excessive gain of potassium might suggest that the muscles were expanded by gaining intracellular fluid. This may be part of the explanation: the second experiment, however, showed that nitrogen was also gained, in about three times the amount expected if the weight gain had been normal muscle.

Table 10.4 *Expected gains of body weight (kg) on methandienone, calculated from observed gains of potassium and of nitrogen, on different assumptions*

Nature of gain	Calculated from	Assumed normal value	Calculated weight gain Exp. 1	Exp. 2
Lean tissue	K	67 mmol/kg	6.3	6.5
Normal muscle	K	90 mmol/kg	4.7	4.8
Intracellular water	K	150 mmol/kg	2.8	2.9
Lean tissue	N	34 g/kg		7.5
Normal muscle	N	31 g/kg		8.3
(Actual weight gain			3.3	2.3)

Interpretation of these changes is hindered by our limited knowledge of the composition of even normal muscle, let alone of the changes brought about by athletic training, drugs, other possibly relevant factors such as diet, and interactions between any of these. The findings might perhaps be explained by postulating gain of protein in the muscle cells together with some of the potassium, but not the phosphate, which normally accompanies it. There would thus be fewer free ions to exert osmotic pressure, and so less than the normal accompaniment of cell fluid. What the functional consequences of this would be it is impossible to say.

Research in the context of meat production may provide some clues to the human situation. Steroids are commonly given to meat animals, though substances described as 'anabolic' in this context are most commonly oestrogens, i.e. analogues of female hormones: substances with male hormone activity are considered ineffective, or effective only when given with oestrogens. The last point parallels our findings in female rats. Meat from treated animals has a markedly changed appearance, with more solid-looking lean and less visible fat; this is the principal reason for the use of steroids. P. J. Buttery and his colleagues have studied the cellular mechanism of action of a male-type steroid, trenbolone acetate, in female animals (Buttery, Vernon, and Pearson, 1978; Vernon and Buttery 1978). They found that the drug reduced the rates of both synthesis and breakdown of muscle proteins; breakdown was slowed most; this led to increased protein content. They suggested that the effect might be brought about through interference with the uptake of glucocorticoids at muscle cells. Glucocorticoids are hormones secreted by the adrenal glands in response to stress. They have a number of actions, which include accelerating the breakdown of cell proteins, making them available as a reserve source of energy. Blocking this action would conserve protein. The studies naturally did not measure muscle performance.

Linèt (1970) has reported evidence of another possible interaction, at liver cells, between anabolic steroids and glucocorticoids. The liver takes up steroids and converts them into inactive compounds; this is the principal means of final disposal of glucocorticoids and anabolic steroids. Linèt found that anabolic steroids appeared to prolong the life of glucocorticoids in the body. Anabolic steroids taken as drugs are present in much greater concentrations in the body than the natural steroids, and it was suggested that they monopolize the uptake mechanisms at the liver cells, so sparing the glucocorticoids.

Table 10.5 shows measurements of hormones made in our first experiment. They are consistent with this concept. Taking methandienone significantly increased the concentration of cortisol (the principal glucorticoid in man) in the blood. It increased the amount excreted unchanged in the urine, i.e. not taken up by the liver. The decreased testosterone concentration also shown implies suppression of secretion of the normal male hormone. This was not surprising; the animal evidence shows that methandienone has androgenic actions, and so it would be expected to interfere with the normal feedback control of testosterone secretion.

There are clues here on which a credible overall explanation of the effects of 'anabolic' steroids can be built up, albeit speculatively (Fig. 10.10). Hard exercise is a sufficient stress to stimulate cortisol secretion. 'Anabolic' steroids taken in large quantities interfere with the uptake of cortisol at the two points shown in Fig. 10.10. At muscles, this leads to slowing of protein breakdown, which produces the expanded, abnormal muscles seen in athletes and (when combined with oestrogen) in steroid-treated meat animals. At the liver it reduces breakdown of cortisol, so increasing the concentration of cortisol in the body. The increase in cortisol concentration may, in the short run, benefit athletes in several ways. It may increase mobilization of energy, increase central nervous arousal, and reduce muscle fatigue. The last effect would enable more work to be done. This may be particularly

Table 10.5 *Measurements of hormones over period on methandienone in experiment 1*

Hormone	Measurement	Start	End	Significance
Cortisol	Concentration in plasma (nmol/l)	290	400	*
Cortisol	Excretion rate in urine (nmol/24 h)	250	450	*
Testosterone	Concentration in plasma (nmol/l)	20	8	**

* 5 per cent,
** 1 per cent level, paired *t* test over period.

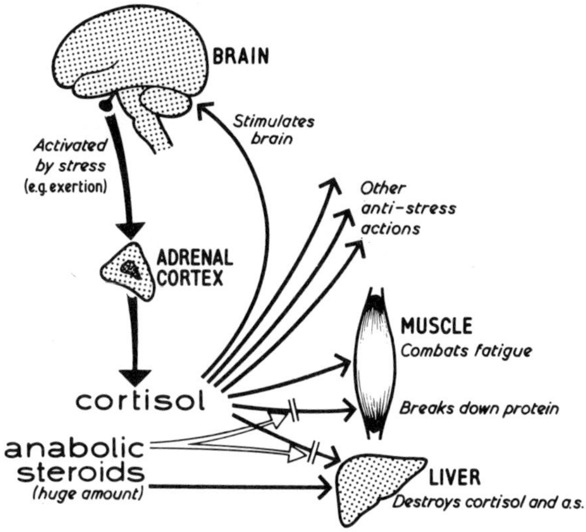

Fig. 10.10. Suggested interaction between anabolic steroids and endogenous cortisol. There is evidence that anabolic steroids block uptake of cortisol at the two points shown. This could account for many of the effects of the drug in athletes.

important during training. It would fit in with the statement some athletes make that steroids are most useful to them during training, simply because they enable more training to be done. This must increase the difficulties of detecting use of steroids.

It has also been suggested that 'anabolic' steroids may have a direct action on the brain, increasing aggressiveness or masking pain. Even in the doses used by athletes, however, they seem to have remarkably little effect on body weight or mental state, in the absence of exertion. This would be consistent with the postulated indirect mechanism of action involving cortisol.

In the long run, taking 'anabolic' steroids in the doses used by athletes seems certain to be harmful. Some of the side-effects are also consistent with the suggested mechanism of action. Excessive production of cortisol occurs in Cushing's disease, where it produces a characteristic puffy appearance of the face and trunk. Long-continued use of 'anabolic' steroids also produces an abnormal appearance, which has at least something in common with that seen in Cushing's disease (Fig. 10.11).

Long-continued suppression of testosterone secretion may eventually become irreversible, and lead to infertility. The long-term consequences of the abnormal composition of the muscles are unknown. Professor V. Wynn has shown that one of the most consistently demonstrable effects of long-term use of 'anabolic' steroids is evidence of damage to the liver (Wynn,

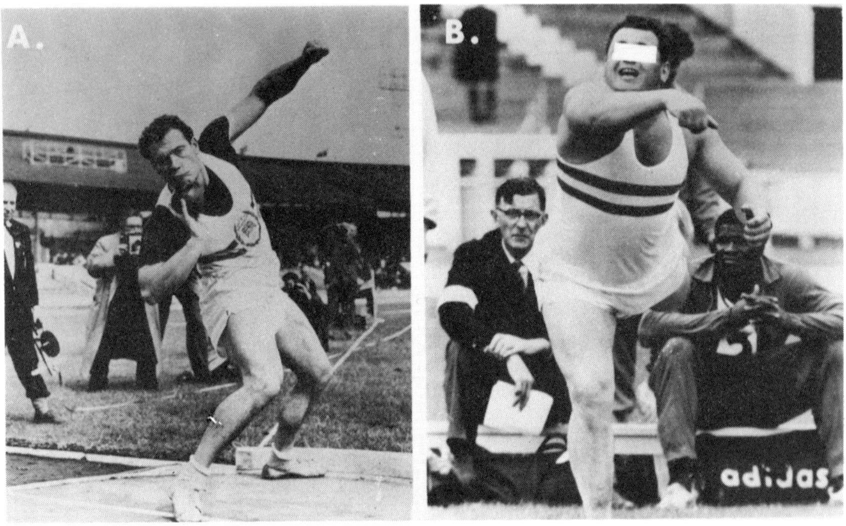

Fig. 10.11. Press photographs of (A) shot putter of the period prior to use of steroids, and (B) discus thrower of more recent period. There seems to have been a consistent change in the appearance of athletes in these events, which *may* be attributable to the use of steroids. (Photographs kindly supplied by Mr W. Poush.)

Landon, and Kawerau 1961). This is presumably connected with the liver's function of disposing of steroids, which may be overloaded. Cancer of the liver has been reported (Johnson, Feagler, Lerner, Majerus, Siegel, Hartmann, and Thomas 1972). Considering the variety and potency of the actions of steroids as a class, however, perhaps the most remarkable thing is

Table 10.6 *Summary of the actions of 'anabolic' steroids in athletes in the light of current evidence*

The size of muscles increases (paralleled in meat animals if oestrogens also present; not seen in inactive rats or (probably) in inactive humans)
Body weight increases
Effect on muscle performance is doubtful
Fatigue may be reduced, and capacity for training increased
The increased bulk of muscles: is *not* normal muscle; is *not* related to the greater weight and muscularity normal in males; *may* be produced by interaction of the drug with endogenous cortisol
Facial and body appearance change
Secretion of testosterone is suppressed
Liver damage occurs eventually

that athletes can consume such large quantities with so little immediate effect.

Table 10.6 summarizes the effects of 'anabolic' steroids in the light of current knowledge.

Acknowledgements

The author gratefully acknowledges the contributions of numerous colleagues, whose names are given in the text or in the list of references, who were full partners in the investigations described; and the patience and co-operation received from the experimental subjects. The Medical Research Council supported part of the investigation, and Ciba-Geigy Ltd. supplied drugs and other assistance.

References

Buttery, P. J., Vernon, B. G., and Pearson, J. T. (1978). Anabolic agents – some thoughts on their mode of action. *Proc. Nutr. Soc.* **37**, 311–15.

Eisenberg, E. and Gordan, G. S. (1950). The levator ani muscle of the rat as an index of myotrophic activity of steroidal hormones. *J. Pharmacol. Exp. Ther.* **99**, 38–44.

Harvey, J. S. (1976). The effects of the gonads on the sex difference in body weight in the rat. M. Phil. thesis, University of Leeds.

—— Hervey, G. R., and Hutchinson, I. (1972). The role of gonadal hormones in determining the sex difference in adult body weight in the rat. *J. Endocrinol.* **57**, xxiv.

Hayes, K. J. (1965). The so-called 'levator ani' of the rat. *Acta Endocrinol. (Copenh.)* **48**, 337–47.

Hervey, E. and Hervey, G. R. (1967). The effects of progesterone on body weight and composition in the rat. *J. Endocrinol.* **37**, 361–84.

—— and Hervey, G. R. (1981). The influence of sex hormones on energy balance. In In *The body weight regulatory system: normal and disturbed mechanisms* (Ed. L. A. Cioffi, W. P. T. James, and T. B. Van Itallie), pp. 345–52. Raven Press, New York.

Hervey G. R. (1969). Regulation of energy balance. *Nature, Lond.* **223**, 629–31.

—— (1975). Are athletes wrong about anabolic steroids? *Br. J. Sports Med.* **9**, 74–7.

—— and Hutchinson, I. (1972). The effects of testosterone on body weight and composition in the rat. *J. Endocrinol.* **57**, xxiv–xxv.

—— —— Knibbs, A. V., Burkinshaw, L., Jones, P. R. M., Norgan, N. G., and Levell, M. J. (1976). 'Anabolic' effects of methandienone in men undergoing athletic training. *Lancet* **2**, 699–702.

—— Knibbs, A. V., Burkinshaw, L., Morgan, D. B., Jones, P. R. M., Chettle, D. R., and Vartsky, D. (1981). Effects of methandienone on the performance and body composition of men undergoing athletic training. *Clin. Sci.* **60**, 457–61.

Hutchinson, I. (1978). The effects of testosterone and 'anabolic' steroids on body weight and composition in the rat. Ph.D. thesis, University of Leeds.

Johnson, F. L., Feagler, J. R., Lerner, K. G., Majerus, P. W., Siegel, M., Hartmann, J. R., and Thomas, E. D. (1972). Association of androgenic–anabolic steroid therapy with development of hepatocellular carcinoma. *Lancet* **2**, 1273–6.

Kochakian, C. D. (1950). Comparison of protein anabolic property of various androgens in the castrated rat. *Am. J. Physiol.* **160**, 53–61.

—— and Murline J. R. (1935). The effect of male hormone on the protein and energy metabolism of castrate dogs. *J. Nutr.* **10**, 437–59.

—— and Tillotson, C. (1957). Influence of several C_{19} steroids on the growth of individual muscles of the guinea pig. *Endocrinology* **60**, 607–18.

—— —— and Endahl, G. L. (1956). Castration and the growth of muscles in the rat. *Endocrinology* **58**, 226–31.

Krüskemper, H. L. (1968). *Anabolic steroids*. Academic Press, New York.

Linèt, O. (1970). Interactions between androgenic–anabolic steroids and glucocorticoids. Fortschr. Arzneimitt Forsch. **14**, 139–95.

Payne, A. H. (1975). Anabolic steroids in athletics. *Br. J. Sports Med.* **9**, 83–8.

Rassaert, C. L., Wolff, A., and McDougall, E. A. (1968). A new technique for extirpation of the levator ani muscle in the rat. *J. Endocrinol.* **42**, 601–2.

Vernon, B. G. and Buttery, P. J. (1978). The effects of trenbolone acetate with time on the various responses of protein synthesis in the rat. *Br. J. Nutr.* **40**, 563–72.

Vida, J. A. (1969). *Androgens and anabolic agents*. Academic Press, New York.

Wynn, V., Landon, J., and Kawerau, E. (1961). Studies of hepatic function during methandienone therapy. *Lancet* **1**, 69–75.

11 Sports science and sports scientists – the athlete's view

P. F. RADFORD

Introduction

Tradition and innovation

Athletes and their coaches have always used whatever is available to help them prepare for their competitions and improve their performance.

New ideas, often untested and unproven, have been eagerly taken up by athletes and mixed in with age-old traditions. Hicks, in 1904, was twice given one sixtieth of a grain of sulphate of strychnine to help him get through the Olympic Marathon; in 1893 William Gunn wore an electropathic belt to improve his strength whilst batting; in 1850 athletes used Dover's Powders, and even earlier, in 1805, ipecacuana and Glauber's Salts were well known ingredients of an athlete's training. In this sense a tension has always existed in the training and preparation for sport; a tension between tradition and innovation, between the old and well-tried methods, and the new way of doing things. However strong the temptation is to stay with what you know, the battle has invariably been won by the forces of change. Athletes have never been content to stay in the pack; almost by definition, they want to be one step ahead. Not surprisingly, therefore, the fashions in training have changed almost as rapidly as haute couture.

As early as the second century AD, Philostratus wrote critically about the modern methods in athletic training, and the dangers of breaking away from traditional methods.

In the continual search for something to give them the edge over the opposition (or to keep up with it), athletes and coaches have listened closely to cranks and charlatans; but have also sieved thoroughly through the ideas of A. V. Hill, Åstrand, and thousands of other scientists: searching the world of science and technology for something, anything, that will expand their knowledge and improve performance.

In this sense athletes and coaches are no different today. Science and sport have never been strangers. What may be different is the potential scope and scale of the effect that science and technology can have on sporting performance.

Sports science is now big business; not the hobby of a few enthusiasts, but the very livelihood of thousands of men and women throughout the world. In some cases sports scientists are almost as well known as the athletes they monitor, and better known than their coaches. Professional sports scientists are seen by many as a new, but essential, part of sport, but little, if anything, is known about the way that athletes view them.

Methods

This paper stems from an attempt to sample athletes' attitudes and opinions towards sports science.

After considerable discussion with athletes, a questionnaire was constructed to sample the attitude and opinions of athletes on the following.

What do athletes think about the quality and quantity of sports scientists today?
What place do athletes think that sports scientists should enjoy in their sport during the next 10 years?
What effect have sports scientists had on their sport?
What effect is sports science likely to have on their sport?
What is the relationship between sports scientists and coaches and athletes, and what is it likely to be in the future?
How can we design a system to deliver sports science knowledge to athletes and coaches?
What aspects of sports science should be given priority in the future?
What areas of sports science do athletes currently use?
What areas of sports science would athletes use if they were available?

What is sports science?

The term 'sports science' is, of course, open to a very wide interpretation, and the label 'sports scientist' may be given by athletes to some with little genuine claim to it. At the start of the questionnaire, therefore, a statement was included which was intended to give guidance to the athletes to help them to interpret these terms. It started by describing the purpose of the questionnaire as an attempt to define the problems and the status of sports science. The introductory statement continued as follows:

> Little is known of what athletes and coaches think of this branch of their sport and it will help me greatly if you would take some time to read through and answer this questionnaire as carefully as possible.
>
> Although there is a space for your name, no names will be used when the results are presented, and I will consider your questionnaire responses to be *strictly confidential.* If you choose not to give your name this, too, is acceptable.
>
> The term *'sports science'* is used to describe the application of scientific methods, knowledge, and principles from any branch of science to sport. This, of course, covers many different types of activity, ranging, for example, from the designing of an aerodynamic javelin to the study of the personality of middle-aged squash players; or from the measurement of the maximum oxygen uptake of an Olympic middle-distance runner to the measurement of the forces produced when performing a back-somersault.

A *'sports scientist'* is, therefore, any person who is knowledgeable in *any* of the disciplines of science who applies his/her knowledge to a sporting problem. There are, unfortunately, many well-meaning, amateur 'experts' in sports science whose expertise would not be generally recognized, and in this questionnaire when I use the term 'sports scientist' I am not referring to these. The term 'sports scientist' in this questionnaire refers to a person who is *knowledgeable, qualified,* and *experienced* in one branch of science and who applies his/her knowledge to sport.

I have kept the questionnaire fairly short so as not to take up too much of your time, but if you have any additional observations to make, please feel free to do so. A space is provided for this purpose at the end of the questionnaire.

Please answer all questions.

Thank you for your help.

The present study achieved a return rate of only eight per cent, and this paper analyses the returns of only 25 athletes who competed at an international level; these were matched with another 25 athletes who compete at a club level only.

The athletes were: British International Track and Field athletes (male and female) with a mean of 5.625 years of international experience. They will be referred to as the International Athletes. British Track and Field athletes (male and female), none of whom had ever been selected to compete at international level. They will be referred to as the Club Athletes.

Replies from athletes from other sports and other nations were collected, but they proved too few to warrant analysis and so are not presented here. Because of the relatively small numbers, this study should be regarded as a pilot study only.

The questionnaire and the subjects

From a large battery of questionnaire items, 17 were selected, which in total required less than 40 responses, and a total time commitment of 10–12 minutes. Items were scattered at random throughout the questionnaire and not presented in sequence on one theme as they are reported here.

Previous experience has shown that athletes do not like completing questionnaires and will avoid doing so whenever possible, and so this questionnaire was kept short, probably too short to explore these issues fully. None of the issues investigated have been treated in depth and much work is required to refine the existing items and to probe further into athletes' opinions.

Keeping the questionnaire short failed, unfortunately, to encourage the co-operation of athletes. Questionnaires were distributed to athletes in the Olympic Village in Moscow, to athletes in training, and to athletes in the stadium on the day of a competition. Some of these places were unlikely to prove popular, but the alternative, that of asking athletes to complete them at home, has proved extremely unsuccessful in the past.

This study, therefore, analyses the responses of 25 experienced international, and 25 club athletes to a series of statements, such as:

During the next 10 years, if coaches are to be successful, they must improve their knowledge of sports sciences.

Scoring

The athletes were required to respond to each statement by selecting one point on a nine-point scale, which corresponded with their attitude to each statement. The nine points ranged from 'very strongly agree' at the one extreme, to 'very strongly disagree' at the other extreme.

These responses will be presented here as mean responses for the group plus the standard error of the mean or standard deviations. To enable these calculations to be made, the following numerical values were given to each of the responses:

Very strongly agree	8.5
Strongly agree	7.5
Moderately agree	6.5
Slightly agree	5.5
Neither agree nor disagree	4.5
Slightly disagree	3.5
Moderately disagree	2.5
Strongly disagree	1.5
Very strongly disagree	0.5

The responses of the two groups (international athletes and club athletes) were compared. An *F* test was used to determine whether the variances of the two groups differed significantly, and the simple Student's *t* test was used to determine whether there was a significant difference between the mean responses of the two groups. With 24 *df* for the larger variance and 24 *df* for the small variance, and *F* value of 1.98 is needed to reject the null hypothesis of no difference between the two group variances at the 0.05 level. An *F* value of 2.66 is needed for the 0.01 level.

When applying Student's *t* test with 48 *df* a value of approximately 2.010 is needed to reject the null hypothesis of no difference between the two group means at the 0.05 level. A *t* value of approximately 2.685 is needed for the 0.01 level and approximately 3.510 for the 0.001 level.

Results

Sports science and sports scientists

Five of the questionnaire items were designed to elicit from the athletes their views on the present and future status of sports science and sports scientists in Britain.

When comparing the two groups of athletes, it was found that for all five items the F values failed to reach 1.98 and so the null hypothesis could not be rejected at even the 0.05 level.

Similarly, for all five items the t values failed to reach 2.010 and so the null hypothesis could not be rejected at even the 0.05 level.

As no significant differences were found in the variances or means of the two groups, the two groups were pooled. British athletes agreed with the following statements about sports science and sports scientists.

The following are the mean responses by the 50 British track and field athletes, plus standard errors of the means. These statements were not arranged in this order in the questionnaire. The item number to the left refers to the number of the item in the questionnaire (see also Fig. 11.1).

8. In Britain there is a need for far more, knowledgeable sports scientists.
   Strongly agree: 7.140 ± 0.301.

13. In Britain there are far fewer knowledgeable sports scientists than in other leading sporting nations.
    Strongly agree: 7.194 ± 0.189.

11. In Britain it is far too difficult to get access to knowledgeable sports scientists.
    Moderately agree: 6.580 ± 0.319.

16. Sports science will play an increasingly important part in sport during the next 10 years.
    Moderately agree: 6.949 ± 0.189.

21. If successes in international competition are to be achieved, sports science will need to play a much more prominent part in Britain during the next 10 years than it does at present.
    Moderately agree: 6.847 ± 0.260.

Interaction between athletes, coaches, and sports scientists

The following four statements all referred to the present and future interaction between athletes, coaches, and sports scientists. As in the previous section the responses of two groups were pooled because no significant differences at the 0.01 level were found on any of the four items between the variances or means of the two groups. Indeed, only in item 9 did the responses reach even the 0.05 level for either test on any item. In this case the F value reached 2.174. The international athletes tended to have the wider range of responses on this item. Means and standard errors of the means of the total group are reported (see also Fig. 11.2).

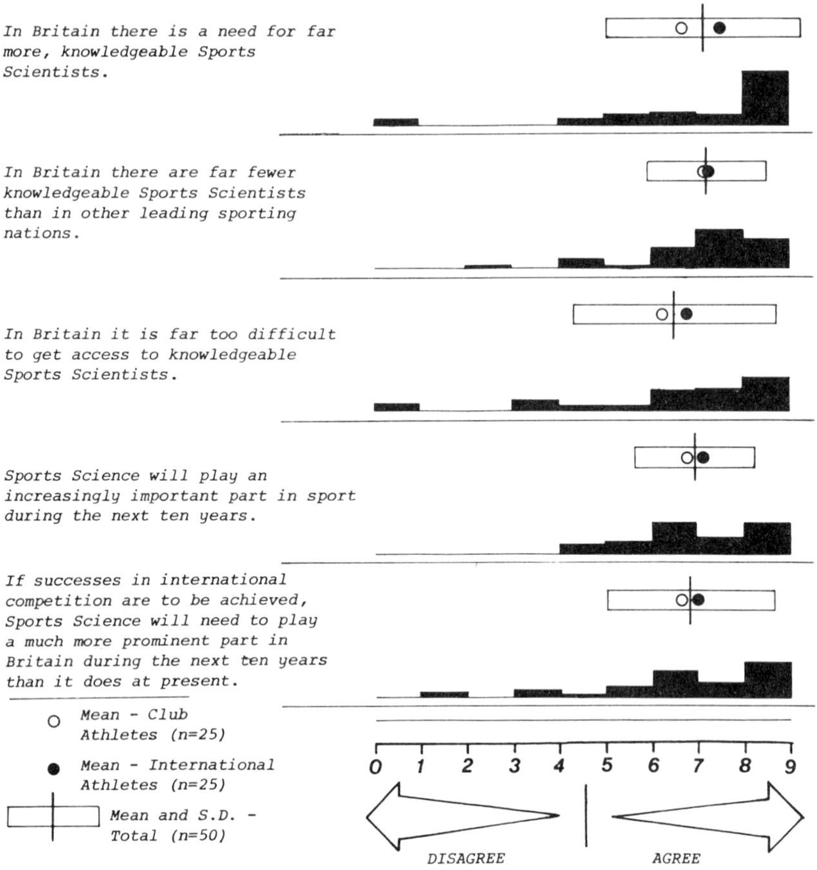

Fig. 11.1. The means, standard deviations and distribution of athletes' responses to statements about Sports Science and Sports Scientists ($n = 50$).

The athletes' mean response was one of moderate disagreement that:

9. Athletes only need to consult or seek advice from sports scientists if their relationship with their coach is not successful.
   Moderately disagree: 2.980 ± 0.287.

Neverthless, there was some agreement with the following:

19. If sports scientists become more influential, their presence will tend to change the nature of the traditional relationship between athletes and their coaches.
    Slightly agree: 5.112 ± 0.324.

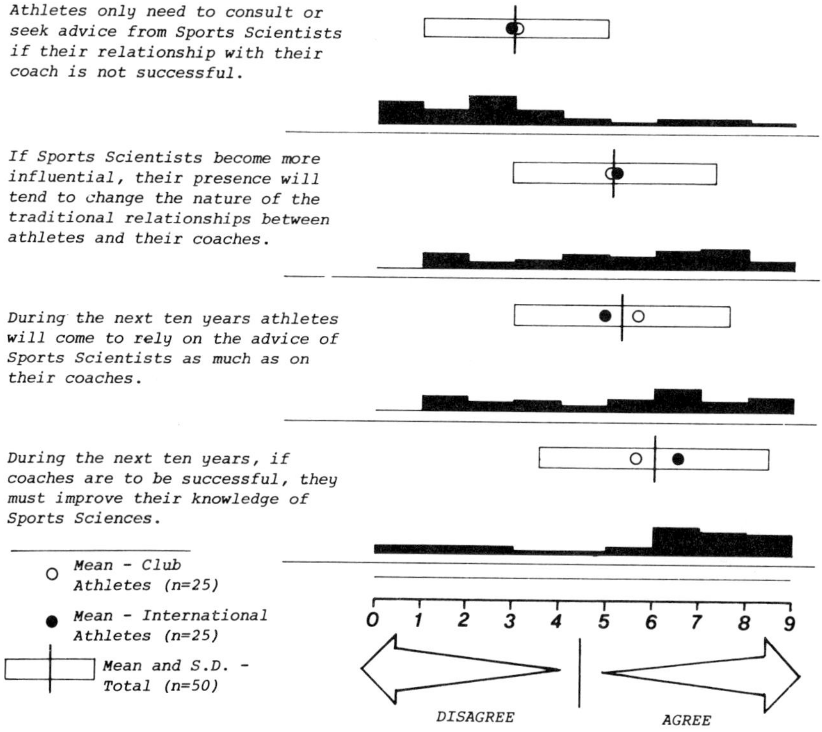

Fig. 11.2. The means, standard deviations and distribution of athletes' responses to statements about the relationships between athletes, coaches, and sports scientists ($n = 50$).

18. During the next 10 years athletes will come to rely on the advice of sports scientists as much as on their coaches.
Slightly agree: 5.296 ± 0.335.

22. During the next 10 years, if coaches are to be successful, they must improve their knowledge of sports sciences.
Moderately agree: 6.042 ± 0.128.

As Fig. 11.2 shows, the dispersion of the athletes' responses is much larger, particularly on items 18 and 19, indicating a much wider divergence of opinion on these statements, than on those of the earlier section, summarized in Fig. 11.1.

Values and ethics of sport

The following four statements all referred to the values and ethics of sport and the effect that the athletes believe sports scientists have and will have on these.

The responses of the club athletes and the international athletes, were pooled because no significant differences at the 0.05 level were found on any of the items between the variances or means of the two groups. Means and standard errors of the means are reported (see also Fig. 11.3).

The athletes' mean response was one of slight disagreement with the statement that:

12. Sports scientists are largely responsible for the unethical developments in modern sport such as the taking of drugs and other substances to improve athletic performance.
    Slightly disagree: 3.625 ± 0.383.

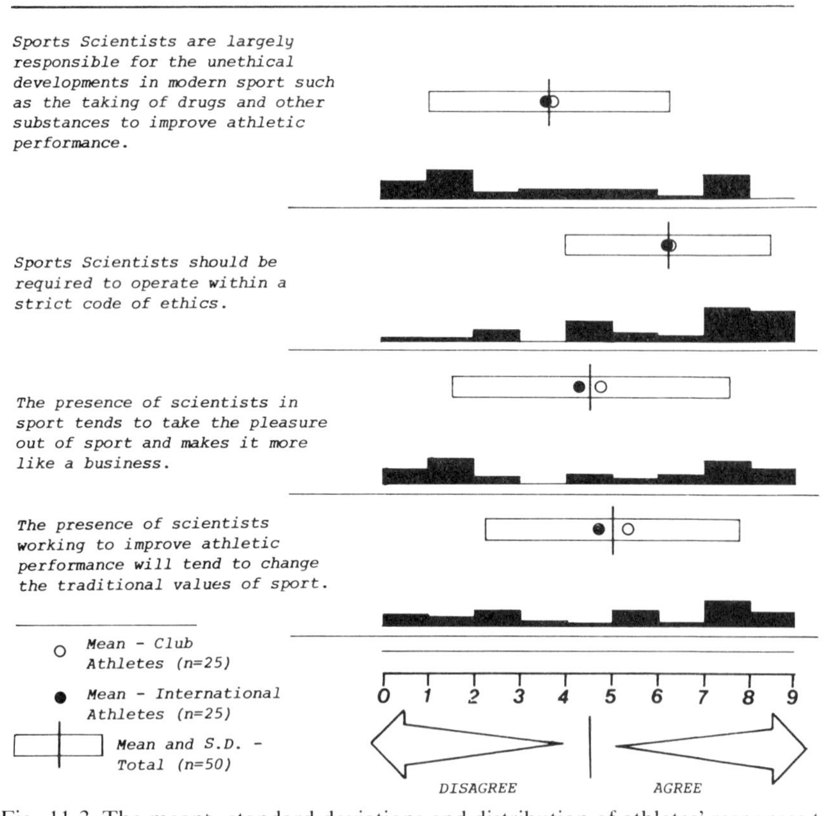

Fig. 11.3 The means, standard deviations and distribution of athletes' responses to statements about the values and ethics of sport and the effects of Sports Science on these (n = 50).

Great caution must be observed in the interpretation of this item because the range of responses was extremely wide. Indeed, there is clear evidence of bi-modality in the athletes' responses. More than two-thirds of all the responses fell into the two most extreme categories at *both* ends of the scale, and although the mean response suggests slight disagreement with the statement that it is the sports scientists who can be held to blame for 'the unethical developments in modern sport', a closer inspection of their answers shows that there are two distinct groups, each of whom hold strong but opposite opinions. Almost 23 per cent of the athletes strongly agreed that the sports scientists were responsible.

Similar care must be exercised in the interpretation of the other three items in this section, for although the mean response shows some agreement with two out of the three statements, the range of scores is very large and there is some evidence of bi-modality in the distribution of scores for all three items, but particularly on 10 and 20 (see Fig. 11.3).

17. Sports scientists should be required to operate within a strict code of ethics.
    Moderately agree: 6.208 ± 0.323.

10. The presence of scientists in sport tends to take the pleasure out of sport and makes it more like a business.
    Neither agree nor disagree: 4.520 ± 0.434.

20. The presence of scientists working to improve athletic performance will tend to change the traditional values of sport.
    Slightly agree: 5.051 ± 0.400.

How funds should be spent

Athletes were also asked to respond to seven statements related to the way that they believe that money should be spent during the next ten years for the development of sports science. Seven potential functions of sports science were listed and they were asked to respond to these seven items on the same nine-point scale as before, but they were additionally asked to remember that if they believed that one function was more important than another, then this should be reflected in their responses. In this way it was hoped to rank the functions in order of the athletes' preference. As previously, the two groups were pooled as their responses were not found to be significantly different.

The means and standard errors of the means for the seven inter-related items are reported below. They are placed in the order of magnitude of their respective means. These seven alternatives were all part of one questionnaire item; the letters (a) to (g) are placed to the left of the statements to indicate their order. See also Fig. 11.4.

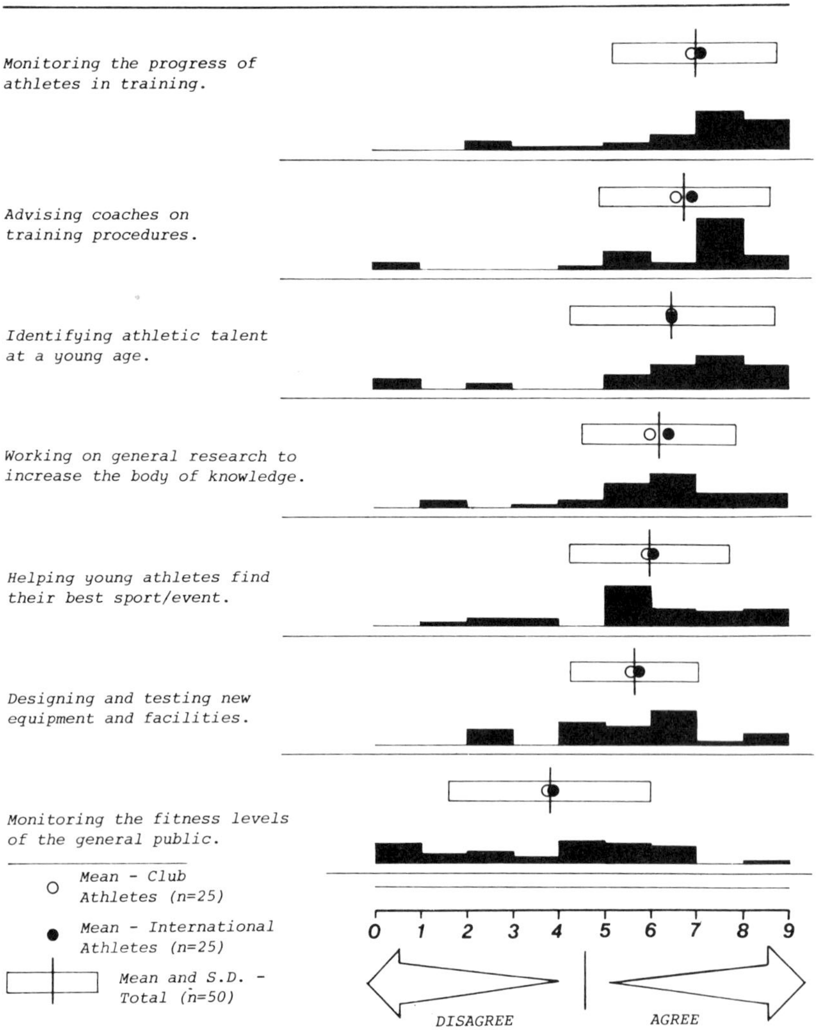

Fig. 11.4. The means, standard deviations and distribution of athletes' responses to statements about the functions of Sports Science that are the most important and should, therefore, be allocated appropriate funds, during the next ten years ($n = 50$).

The order that emerged was as follows:

1st (b) Monitoring the progress of athletes in training.
Strongly agree: 7.000 ± 0.245.

2nd (c) Advising coaches on training procedures.
Moderately agree: 6.740 ± 0.266.

3rd (a) Identifying athletic talent at a young age.
Moderately agree: 6.500 ± 0.314.

4th (g) Working on general research to increase the body of knowledge.
Moderately agree: 6.200 ± 0.238.

5th (d) Helping young athletes find their best sport/event.
Moderately agree: 6.040 ± 0.246.

6th (e) Designing and testing new equipment and facilities.
Slightly agree: 5.640 ± 0.206.

7th (f) Monitoring the fitness levels of the general public.
Slightly disagree: 3.820 ± 0.315.

As before, caution must be used when interpreting the responses ranked third and seventh, as in both cases there was an extremely wide scatter of responses. For example, although the largest number (20 per cent) neither agree nor disagree that sports scientists should monitor the fitness levels of the general public, an equal number share the two most extreme responses at either end of the scale; the mean response therefore tells only part of the story.

The athletes were also asked about the future development and funding of sports science. They were asked to rank in order the agencies that they would prefer to see handling the funds for, and the administration of, sports science. This questionnaire item proved to be unsuitable for its purpose, and the following analysis is based also on the often lengthy comments added by the athletes. Responses of the international athletes only are reported here.

The rank ordering of the agencies was as follows:

1st – Universities and colleges;
2nd – National governing bodies of sport;
3rd – Sports Council;
4th – Government;
5th – Private industry;
6th – Local sports clubs;
7th – Local government.

These alternatives are not, of course, mutually exclusive. Delivering the knowledge of sports science to those who will use it may require several agencies working in concert. The following arrangement seems to get the strongest support.

> Money made available to the Sports Council from Government sources should then, on the advice of the national governing bodies of sport, be

passed on to specified universities and colleges who would be responsible for completing the work they have been contracted to perform.

Athletes favour the money coming mainly from the Government but not administered by it (they may have thought differently if the questionnaires had been completed before the Moscow Olympic Games), but, in the opinion of the athletes neither private industry, local clubs, nor local government have any effective part to play in the development or administration of sports science within the next 10 years.

The branches of sports science

Athletes were also asked whether they had consulted or been advised during the previous 12 months by someone, other than their coach, with specialist knowledge in any of six branches of sports science. They were also asked which areas they needed or would have liked specialist advice on during the same period time had it been available. International athletes and club athletes are listed separately, their responses being summarized in Table 11.1.

Table 11.1 indicates that only with sports injuries do the British international athletes surveyed receive the care or advice they are seeking. The same is true of the club athletes. The large number of athletes of all levels who require help with sports injuries in the course of a year must give concern, and almost certainly deserves closer scrutiny.

The list in Table 11.1 is not, of course, complete, and athletes were invited to add to it.

Some athletes at all levels wanted information and advice on injury prevention.

Some athletes at all levels wanted access to medical practitioners who

Table 11.1. *Number (expressed as a percentage) of athletes consulting or seeking advice from six branches of sports science during the previous 12 months*

	Did consult		Would have consulted if available	
	International athletes	Club athletes	International athletes	Club athletes
Exercise physiology	12	12	74	64
Biomechanics	16	12	61	68
Sports psychology	16	16	67	56
Motor learning/performance	12	12	56	72
Sports injuries	84	76	84	100
Nutrition	32	28	79	88

could give advice on when to return to full training after minor illnesses (e.g., influenza, diarrhoea, nausea).

Some international athletes expressed a desire to consult with a pharmacologist.

Discussion

The questionnaire responses from athletes of all abilities tended, in some cases, to do no more than confirm the predictable. This is not in itself a bad thing – for example, no one working in the world of British sport at this time would expect anything other than for athletes to agree that there are fewer knowledgeable sports scientists in Britain than in other leading sporting nations. What is surprising, perhaps, is that this statement would elicit the most extreme response of all the items in the questionnaire. Does this suggest some form of mild paranoia in our athletes? Certainly I detected from many athletes the feeling that they (British athletes) were worse off than others and that this was somehow unfair. With some international athletes this seemed to go as far as to suggest a sense of persecution, but perhaps this was a reaction to the unique political and social pressures centred on the Moscow Olympic Games that were present when the questionnaires were completed.

Within the athletes' responses are many suggestions and implications for the coaches, the sports scientists, and the administrators of the sport, some of which may be helpful to them as they plan for the future.

In general, British track and field athletes feel that in Britain there are too few sports scientists and that it is too difficult to gain access to those there are. In addition, they believe that in the next ten years sports science is likely to become even more important than it is today.

Athletes seem to view their preparation as involving a three-way partnership involving themselves, their coaches, and sports scientists. But coaches, be warned – athletes think that in the future you will need to improve your knowledge of the sports sciences. In addition, you must learn to adapt to a situation in which your athletes may rely on the advice from sports scientists as much as from yourself.

If athletes are willing to welcome a new form of partnership involving the sports scientists, their coaches, and themselves, there will be many coaches and scientists equally willing, I am sure.

Nevertheless, sports scientists in particular must be aware of their image. Despite the varied response from athletes, one in three athletes did agree that the sports scientists were responsible for the unethical developments in modern sport, such as drug taking. This does not suggest that even these believed the sports scientists were entirely responsible, nor does it suggest who is. Any attempt to find a single culprit is likely to be misleading, and it is probably in the complex interplay of athletes' and coaches' ambitions, developing technology, and political and/or social pressure that we are likely to find the reasons for these undesirable developments.

There is, among some athletes, however, an undisguised amorality about their approach to sport and sports science, and this I found worrying. One athlete commented:

> I am only interested in sports scientists if they can give me an advantage over other athletes.

Another wrote:

> Athletes will use whatever methods are available – the sports scientist should check to see it is done safely.

Another wrote that:

> They (the sports scientists) should only be concerned with the pure science – the morals are the business of athletes and coaches.

I hope that few sports scientists or administrators would agree with that, and I would be surprised if the majority of sports scientists, coaches, and others did not agree that it is not only the sports scientists who should operate within a strict code of ethics!

There seems to be no doubt in the minds of athletes that sports scientists can improve performance, but are there some circumstances when they should not? Are there some methods that should not be used? On these difficult questions the athletes can give us no help – they too are divided.

If using amphetamines or anabolic steroids is cheating, is improving strength by electric stimulation, or improving $\dot{V}O_{2\,max}$ by altitude training also cheating? What about hypnosis, glycogen loading, blood boosting, eleutherococcus, and testosterone?

It seems that the sports scientists must be aware of their image in more than one way: by bringing new possibilities for improving performance, they change the existing values of sport and in some people's minds the sports scientist is seen as an agent of temptation! But some of the athletes' responses suggest something equally sinister, and that is that the very presence of sports scientists spoils sport! Athletes were almost equally divided over whether the presence of scientists in sport tends to take the pleasure out of it and make it more like a businesss. Most athletes, however, tended to take extreme views, 36 per cent strongly or very strongly agreed with this view, 38 per cent strongly or very strongly disagreed.

Nevertheless, it must be disconcerting to the sports scientists that one in three athletes in this study held such a jaundiced view of them and their role. What can sports scientists have done to provoke such a reaction? The answer is probably that it is not what they have done, but what they represent. Among the range of reasons why some people engage in sport is that they are searching for fun, enjoyment, or self-satisfaction, although it is fashionable, at present, to ridicule such motives. It is unlikely that sports scientists will address themselves to the problems of adding to an athlete's fun, as wholeheartedly as they might address themselves to something more tangible, such as improving their performance. There have always been athletes and coaches whose exclusive goals have been improved performance, prestige, or recognition, and for them the process of involvement in the sport is less important than the end-product. Some athletes, particularly the club athletes, feel that by focussing on the measurable end-product of improved performance sports science will tip the balance away from fun to drudgery, and to them the very presence of sports scientists is alarming.

Let us all hope, however, that the cynicism of one club athlete is found to be groundless; he wrote that:

> Sports scientists can only serve to accelerate the trend towards politicization and professionalization of sport. . . . Sports science seems to have little part to play in the development of a healthy society which keeps sport in its rightful place – as a pastime.

This view may not be typical of the modern elite athlete, but there is enough support for it from the athletes' questionnaire responses to suggest that the tensions between traditional values and new methods that have been present in sport for centuries will continue to be with us for a long time to come.

Acknowledgements

My sincere thanks are offered to those athletes who took the time to complete the questionnaire, so many of whom entered into the spirit of it by adding detailed notes to explain or expand on their responses. I would also like to thank all those officials who helped by distributing and collecting the questionnaires.

12 The future of sports science: a 'brave new world' indeed

R. J. SHEPHARD

To speak of 'the future of sports science' highlights the current dilemma of athlete and academic alike – many sports are rapidly becoming precise hand-maidens of science, with all the limitations of human artistry and creativity implied by such a development. By way of example, the New York Academy of Sciences was able to assemble an impressive 1000 page monograph on marathon running (Milvy 1977), and a series of four international meetings has facilitated collection of at least an equal volume of information on swimming (Eriksson and Fürberg 1978). The eager doctoral student who wishes to establish his reputation by exploring new frontiers of knowledge must select one of the more obscure sports such as dinghy sailing (Niinimaa, Wright, Shephard, and Clarke 1977) or white-water paddling (Sidney and Shephard 1973) where there remain no more than perhaps ten scientific papers in the world literature.

What importance should we attach to this quest for numerical wisdom? Must the athlete and the coach master this mass of new data? Must the physical educator justify his existence by joining a headstrong pursuit for further facts and figures? Among my colleagues in Toronto, there are still philosophers and historians who speak nostalgically of sports studies rather than sports sciences. With all the bravado of Don Quixote, they tilt at Auguste Comte's windmills of positivism, extolling the virtues of a metaphysical and even a theological approach to human activity (Braaten 1978). Fortunately, a humanistic and even a contemplative approach to sport and society remains possible within the relative security of our ivory towers (Whitson 1978). But in the external world of super-powers and stadia there seems little time for contemplation. The scramble is to assemble a sufficiency of scientific facts, on the assumption that one's rival will then be out-performed, justifying on a cost/benefit scale of values expenditures that have been made in the preparation and support of international competitors.

The quest is for knowledge (or as the scientist prefers to call it, information) rather than beliefs and values (Shephard 1974a). A similar progression (or as my humanist colleagues might argue, a similar regression) can be traced in other disciplines. The Hippocratic physician discussed health in terms of an inner harmony of man's vital humours. Medical philosophers were content to paint pictures of disease – chlorosis, plethora, and fever. But with the natural evolution of medicine such picturesque descriptions were displaced by more precise semantic information – anaemia, hypertension, and raised body temperature. These terms have in turn given way to selective information – normally distributed, digital variables that can be manipulated by a computer – a haemoglobin concentration, a blood pressure reading, and an oral or a rectal temperature.

In medicine, selective information is fast displacing intuitive clinical acumen; the machine can often out-perform the physician in both diagnosis and treatment. In other areas of knowledge, evolution is less advanced. Measurement of height, weight, skinfold thicknesses, hip, and breast dimensions can scarcely determine even the external beauty of a woman. Likewise, the sports scientist has far to travel before his measurements can be translated into an unequivocal index of a graceful performance. Many of the variables that apparently influence competitive success, such as skill and personality, have scarcely moved beyond the stage of picturesque description. But given the technical capability of modern microprocessors, such items of information may well be placed on a firm selective basis within our lifetime.

The philosopher enjoys a little uncertainty in human performance. Indeed, social psychologists tell us that the element of 'chance' is an important motive for sports participation (Kenyon 1968). But the name of the game in government-supported and government-dominated laboratories is a ruthless determinism. Every aspect of the athlete's performance is being translated into numbers, with the hope that an appropriate statistical method of combining this information will identify the superstars. Present knowledge of some sports has already reached the point where laboratory measurements can predict the relative ranking of competitors under relaxed conditions. Although resisted by many athletes, laboratory selection procedures have some advantages; objective scores offer a counterpoint to a biased coach, and with some simplification could facilitate a national search for youngsters well-endowed for specific types of competition. Nevertheless, the accuracy of prediction methods is limited at present, and test scores may give a misleading indication of how an individual will perform under the stress of a major international competition (Shephard 1978).

I suspect that time and the microprocessor will overcome this current limitation of sports science. We will discover how to distinguish the competitor who will be spurred to new heights of performance under the gaze of an Olympic crowd, and how to pick out the performer who will 'choke' at the crucial moment. A situation can indeed be envisaged where prediction procedures will become so precise that the expense and tensions of an international competition are no longer necessary. Uncertainty will be reduced until the outcome of an event can be predicted with the required accuracy simply by feeding an agreed series of automated physiological, biochemical, biomechanical, and psychological scores into a well-programmed computer. If you rebel against what seems an Orwellian vision of sports science, may I remind you that the passage of a mere 30 years made many aspects of *Nineteen eighty four* all too true. We should indeed borrow from the insight of another twentieth-century prophet, Aldous Huxley, and foresee the moment when the system is slammed into reverse-gear, the production-line of developing citizens being progressively reprogrammed to ensure that the output meets the aspirations of the sports scientist's computer. The cradle-snatching of some Eastern European sports institutes ominously heralds the 'Brave New World' of the seventh century After Ford, a time when we have learnt to control the human assembly line from the earliest moment after hatching of the ovum. Sperm banks contributed by ageing gold medallists will finally break the genetic barrier. Subsequent control of growth and development will ensure the maturation of individuals totally matched to their athletic destiny, willing to pursue the objectives of sports bureaucrats with the ruthless efficiency of robots.

It is a disturbing prospect. Undoubtedly, future generations of sports scientists will be faced by moral dilemmas that will make current controversies, such as the use of steroids and blood-doping, seem innocent diversions. Rather than attempt to chart details of the course the sports scientist should follow through the dangerous waters of this new knowledge (Shephard 1976a), it seems preferable to discuss the axiology of the voyage. What are the ethical responsibilities of an investigator, and what tactics will be most effective in maintaining acceptable values in a rapidly changing world?

The traditional British appeal has been to fair play and sportsmanship. This approach may have worked when games were played in the circumscribed milieu of Matthew Arnold and Charles Kingsley, but it has little relevance for the sports scientist who lives in a world where many of the competitors and their coaches have not even heard of 'muscular Christianity'. It presupposes operation within an absolute code of moral values; standards of behaviour stem from a particular form of religious belief, and are enforced because they have become the socially accepted norm.

A second possible posture sometimes discussed is a systematic attempt to halt the progress of knowledge, or at least to modify its evolutionary course. Analogies of this tactic exist in other branches of learning, where scientists have for ethical reasons refused to carry out research on nuclear fission, and on materials of potential interest for chemical and biological warfare. It must be immediately admitted that such protests have had little influence upon the course of history – most major nations now have their arsenal of atomic weapons, and the rejection of chemical and biological warfare has stemmed from a recognition of its limited effectiveness rather than from the moral scruples of the scientists involved. In the sports sciences, individual investigators have favoured progress towards more esoteric topics such as the influence of physical activity upon subcellular structure; in contrast, governmental supporting agencies have made increasingly strident demands for 'applied' research, seeking data that has instant reference to problems of athletic performance. Some workers continue to reject tempting research grants for the study of steroids or blood doping, but inevitably others with differing perceptions of values take their place. Our chances of stemming the tide of scientific knowledge are no greater than those of Canute as he faced an advancing ocean. The sports scientist, like his contemporary in any other discipline, must accept as inevitable displacement of the semantic by the selective, with exponential growth of the latter type of information. Nor is this growth an evil to be regretted. In the absence of knowledge, bias, bigotry, and frank charlatanism flourish; a similar situation existed in the natural sciences 500 years ago, and in the biological sciences 150 years ago. In certain of the sports disciplines, there are still charlatans, and only further knowledge can chase away such exploiters of the sportsman and the public purse.

In the specific context of doping control, a third tactic adopted by the earnest investigator has been to claim that the proposed procedure either is ineffective or has an adverse effect upon human performance (Williams 1974). Superficially, this seemed an attractive approach to the older generation of sports scientists, since available evidence suggested that most of the available ergogenic aids did not improve performance. However, in practice a number of problems arose. The athlete did not always accept the word of the scientist – indeed, if he was under the spell of a charlatan, it was sometimes hinted that the scientist was jealous, out-of-date, or unfamiliar with the virtues of the latest wonder drug. In any event, it proved discouraging work for the scientist; his time became devoted to a series of negative investigations, as he sought to counter every wild hypothesis that was advanced. A substantial pool of subjects was needed to ensure that the absence of effect was a genuine finding rather than a statistical artefact (the beta, or type 2 error). A double-blind protocol had to be sustained in the face of curious subjects who were prepared to break open capsules and even submit drugs for chemical analysis (Shephard, Stuart, Campbell, Wright, and Pimm 1974); belief in the efficacy of a drug sometimes had as large an effect upon performance as its true pharmacological action. When the research was finally completed, it remained difficult to arrange for the publication of negative results, so that there was a danger that both athletes and scientific colleagues would remain unaware that a given drug or procedure was of no benefit to a competitor.

In any event, the value of the technique has lessened, since there is now a real danger that effective procedures are being discovered. It is hard not to believe that the intense muscle development seen in a pubertal boy is causally related to an increased output of male sex hormones. Experimental opinion on the response to synthetic androgens remains divided, but some apparently well-designed animal studies have shown an increase of muscle mass when well-fed and well-trained animals have been given anabolic steroids (American College of Sports Medicine 1977). In man, considerations of safety have limited experiments to much smaller doses of drugs than those ingested by some athletes. There is agreement that the anabolic steroids increase body mass. Some authors have attributed this phenomenon to water retention, but other investigators have observed a true increase of lean tissue, along with an increase of appetite and an augmentation of competitiveness. Certainly, few athletes accept scientific statements that anabolic steroids have no influence upon muscle development, and many competitors are convinced that they cannot reach international standards except by use of such drugs.

In several other areas of physiological manipulation, negative results are now being traced to faults of experimental technique rather than an absence of benefit. Blood doping, for example, will augment performance, but only if adequate precautions are taken to conserve the vitality of the red cells (Gledhill, Buick, Froese, Spriet, and Meyers 1978). Hypnosis will increase muscular strength (Ikai and Steinhaus 1961), oxygen inhalation will enhance both brief performance and recovery rates (Shephard 1977), altitude training sometimes boosts endurance for at least a short period (Shephard 1974b), and selective patterns of nerve stimulation, or neural doping, may facilitate conversion of muscle fibres from Type IIa, the variety that can handle only sprinting activity, to Type IIb, fibres with both oxidative and glycogen splitting potency (Taylor, Kots, and Lavoie 1978). Even transcendental meditation is being exploited with apparent success as a preliminary to competition. The sports scientist thus can no longer honestly claim there are no physiological and pharmacological tricks to gain an unfair advantage over a rival performer – full exploitation of scientific knowledge already gives a substantial edge to the laboratory-directed competitor, and this margin will increase rapidly over the next few years.

An alternative tactic has been to suggest that the proposed manipulation of the athlete is unsafe. Attention has been focused on the addictive properties of certain stimulants and the risk of death from over-heating of the body when amphetamines are used by distance competitors (Shephard 1976b). Stress has been placed upon the dangers of hypnosis and other forms of mind control. In particular, there is substantial continuing interest in side-effects of the anabolic steroids, including premature closure of epiphyses, liver damage, masculinization of the female competitor, and inhibition of normal hormone secretion by the pituitary hypophysis (American College of Sports Medicine 1977; Shephard, Killinger, and Fried 1977). While it is right that the sports scientist should have the fullest knowledge of these dangers, and should be in a position to warn the athlete against them, too often he is manipulated into the role of an accomplice. For example, an athlete may tell an endocrinologist that he knows all the dangers of using an anabolic compound, and would like regular sperm counts and hormone assays so that he can decide when to stop self-administration of the drug. The glamour of international success and professional salaries (or their equivalent in Eastern European terms) persuade many performers that the prospect of permanent damage to the body is an acceptable risk.

The current weapon of the International Olympic Committee is a complex system of doping controls. In essence, this is an attempt to enforce an external system of values upon the athletes. This approach has apparently had a reasonable measure of success in reducing usage of easily-detected drugs such as the amphetamines (Dirix 1978). However, to many people policing merely adds to the excitement of a contest, and a variety of ingenious ruses have been adopted to foil the control system; officials have detected a switching of urine samples, the hiding of 'clean' urine in a plastic bag under the arm pit, and deliberate manipulation of the volume and acidity of the urine. A further difficulty with formal controls is that many of the apparently more effective types of treatment defy external detection. How can a judge obtain conclusive proof of nerve-doping, hypnosis, or other forms of psychological conditioning? Is there any unequivocal method of deciding that a competitor has recently received a transfusion of his own stored blood? Modern combinations of gas chromatography and mass spectroscopy allow a distinction to be drawn between natural and synthetic steroids (Kochakian 1976), but testing can be made ineffective by a change in the acidity of the urine. Furthermore, anabolic drugs are only detectable for 1–2 days, while their effects persist for weeks, if not months. Officials hope to catch more flagrant violations through random spot-checks of urine in athletes showing a suspiciously large increase of body mass. Nevertheless, it seems likely that competitors who wish to flout the rules will find some method of keeping one pace ahead of enforcement agencies with steroid administration as with other forms of doping.

Sports politics (Kidd 1978) is an interesting sub-discipline of sports sociology that has shown vigorous growth of late. The investigators concerned have sensed the exploitation of the athlete and the pressure to unfair methods of competition as an almost inevitable consequence of the politicization of sport. The games of classical Greece were marked by the Pax Olympica, and were in a sense a religious rite, the athlete expressing in the Olympic Oath a sense of spiritual preparedness and an inner feeling of devotion to an ideal greater than himself. Baron de Coubertin cherished these same ideals in re-establishing the Games. His speeches continually stressed the search for physical beauty and health through a happy balance of mind and body, and the value of sport in promoting social democracy and international understanding. 'Dishonour would not lie in defeat, but in failure to take part' (Carl Diem Institute 1966). But current contests assume the pattern of a 'Bellum Olympica'. How serious is this for our society? In the short-term, an Olympic war is less costly and less destructive than a shooting war; however, in the long-term it may cause at least equal damage. Political ideologies and beliefs are becoming accepted not on their intrinsic merits, but rather on their ability to push athletic representatives to the fore by fair means or foul. Whereas classical warfare was marked by an occasional redeeming episode of valour, the present generation of warrior-athletes are in danger of becoming sub-human puppets in a battle waged by technologists from the safety of government-supported laboratories. Further, the battle spectacle is carried into every home by television, the charade of sportsmanship and judging being applauded by an increasingly partial public. Who is to say that in the long-term this mass erosion of social values may not have more ominous consequences for civilization than a nuclear holocaust? One remedy proposed by some of the more thoughtful athletes is a depoliticization of the Games. Each competitor would appear not as a national warrior, but as a humble individual. Whether such a proposal would be accepted by those with vested interests in the present system, and whether the public could divorce the individual performance from the national origin of the competitor, remains problematical.

Although I am a natural optimist, I doubt that any of the simple remedies we have discussed will check the current trend towards total control of the bodies and minds of high-performance athletes. Knowledge provided by the sports scientist will be ruthlessly exploited from the moment of selection in early childhood until the ultimate appearance on the victor's platform. Such an evolution of applied science is currently programmed to occur, despite reactions ranging from indifference to abhorrence on the part of individual athletes and investigators. The only path of escape from this bleak future lies through a fuller development of beliefs and values by the competitor and the laboratory worker alike.

For the competitor and his sponsors to focus strictly upon the measurable variables of the 'hard' sciences such as physiology and biochemistry is to deny the essential nature of his humanity. Even if the prime goal is performance, at the great moments of athletic history this is determined as much by self-concept and internal rewards as by any tangible factor of environment or physiology (Maslow 1962). Indeed, there is a cumulative interaction between self-concept and performance. If an athlete realizes that he has performed well, this enhances his self-image, and increases the prospect of future victories. Real greatness is unlikely to evolve where a competitor sees himself simply in the terms of the scientist – an exciting oxygen-transport system with maximum glycogen-loading of his functional cells.

The investigator does not need to retreat from 'hard' science – this can broaden his understanding of the human condition and suggest fascinating new hypotheses. But there is a real challenge to reestablish the traditional unity of science and philosophy – to ensure that all of our Doctors of Philosophy are indeed philosophers eager to translate new information not only into physical performance, but also into beliefs and values. Much of the current unhealthy abuse of new knowledge could be avoided if it were freely available to all sports scientists and coaches. Meetings such as the one which gave rise to this collection of papers play an important role in this regard, but there is still too much secrecy and 'classified' information. At the University of Toronto, we have a firm rule that no research contract may be accepted unless there is an unconditional guarantee that the resulting data may be published in the world literature. Given universal adoption of this policy, there would be little scope for governments to exploit the research of the sports scientist in their attempts to gain an unfair national advantage.

An even more important step is for us to recognize that contests will remain unequal. One man is big, another small. One represents a national population of 800 million, another a country of eight million people. The ultimate reward of the athlete must be the knowledge that he or she has achieved personal perfection – dishonour is not in defeat, but in failure to participate. This is a hard lesson for any competitor to learn. Perhaps one application of our current sophisticated technology will be to show an individual his own potential, and to assist him in achieving this personal victory.

References

American College of Sports Medicine (1977). Position statement on the use and abuse of anabolic-androgenic steroids in sports. *Med. Sci. Sports* **9**, xi–xiii.

Braaten, C. E. (1978). Theology and the body. In *Physical activity and human well-being*, (eds. F. Landry and W. A. R. Orban) pp. 313–22. Symposia Specialists, Miami, Fla.

Carl Diem Institute (1966). *The Olympic Idea*. Carl Diem Institute, Cologne.

Dirix, A. (1978). Examens anti-doping effectués in 1975 par la ligue vélocipédique belge. In *Sports medicine*. (eds. F. Landry and W. A. R. Orban, pp. 301–5. Symposia Specialists, Miami, Fla.

Eriksson, B. and Fürberg, B. (1978). *Swimming medicine IV*. University Park Press, Baltimore, Md.

Gledhill, N., Buick, F. J., Froese, A. B., Spriet, L. and Meyers, E. C. (1978). An optimal method of storing blood for blood boosting. *Med. Sci. Sports* **10**, 10.

Ikai, M. and Steinhaus, A. H. (1961). Some factors modifying the expression of human strenth. *J. appl. Physiol.* **16**, 157–63.

Kenyon, G. S. (1968). Six scales for assessing attitude toward physical activity. *Res. Q.* **39**, 566–74.

Kidd, B. (1978). *The political economy of sport*. Canadian Association for Health, Physical Education, and Recreation, Ottawa.

Kochakian, C. D. (1976). *Anabolic–androgenic steroids*, pp. 1–725. Springer Verlag, Berlin.
Maslow, A. (1962). *Towards a psychology of being*. Van Nostrand, Princeton, NJ.
Milvy, P. (1977). The marathon: physiological, medical, epidemiological and psychological studies. *Ann. N.Y. Acad. Sci.* **301**, 1–1090.
Niinimaa, V., Wright, G., Shephard, R. J. and Clarke, J. (1977). Characteristics of the successful dinghy sailor. *J. Sports Med. Phys. Fitness* **17**, 83–96.
Shephard, R. J. (1974a). Men at work. *Applications of ergonomics to performance and design*. Thomas. Springfield, Ill.
—— (1974b). Altitude training camps. *Br. J. Sports Med.* **8**, 38–45.
—— (1976a). Sports medicine – new perspectives. *Can. J. appl. Sports Sci.* **1**, 119–22.
—— (1976b). Environment and sports medicine. In *Sports medicine* (eds. J. P. G. Williams and P. Sperryn) Butterworths, London.
—— (1978). The prediction of athletic performance by laboratory and field tests – an overview. In *Physical fitness assessment*, (Eds. R. J. Shephard and H. Lavallée) pp. 113–41. Thomas, Springfield, Ill.
—— (1979). *Endurance fitness*. 2nd edn. University of Toronto Press. Toronto.
—— Killinger D., and Fried, T. (1977). Responses to sustained use of anabolic steroid. *Br. J. Sports Med.* **11**, 170–3.
—— Stuart, D., Campbell, R., Wright, G., and Pimm, P. (1974). Do athletes need vitamin E? *Phys Sports Med.* **2**, 57–60.
Sidney, K. H. and Shephard, R. J. (1973). Physiological characteristics of the whitewater paddler. *Int. Z. angew. Physiol.* **31**: 1–17.
Taylor, A. W., Kots, Y. M. and Lavoie, M. (1978). The effects of faradic stimulation on skeletal muscle fibre area. *Can. J. appl. Sports Sci.* **3**, 185.
Whitson, D. J. (1978). *Research methodology in sport sociology*. Canadian Association for Health, Physical Education and Recreation, Ottawa.
Williams, M. H. (1974). *Drugs and athletic performance*. Thomas, Springfield, Ill.

Index